DRUGS AND SPORTS

Other Books in the At Issue Series:

DRUGS AND SPORTS

William Dudley, *Book Editor*

David L. Bender, *Publisher*
Bruno Leone, *Executive Editor*

Bonnie Szumski, *Editorial Director*
Stuart B. Miller, *Managing Editor*

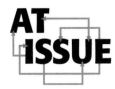

An Opposing Viewpoints® Series

Greenhaven Press, Inc.
San Diego, California

Library of Congress Cataloging-in-Publication Data

Drugs and sports / William Dudley, book editor.
       p.   cm. — (At issue)
   Includes bibliographical references and index.
   ISBN 1-56510-696-2 (pbk. : alk. paper) —
ISBN 1-56510-697-0 (lib. : alk. paper)
   1. Doping in sports. I. Dudley, William. II. Series: At issue
(San Diego, Calif.)

RC1230 .D783   2001
362.29—dc21   00-059632
                                                  CIP

Table of Contents

Introduction

One of the most exciting sports stories in recent years was the attempt to break Roger Maris's single-season home run record in baseball. On September 8, 1998, Mark McGwire of the St. Louis Cardinals made history by hitting his sixty-second home run. The popular McGwire, who finished the season with seventy home runs, was widely celebrated for his feat.

However, many people believe that McGwire's achievement was tarnished by a revelation some weeks earlier that he had been using androstenedione, a compound that temporarily boosts levels of the male sex hormone testosterone. "Andro" is believed by some to promote muscle buildup and recovery; McGwire had taken it as part of his power lifting exercise regimen. It is legal to buy androstenedione as a "dietary supplement" in the United States, although many medical experts believe it is essentially similar to artificial forms of testosterone (steroids) that are illegal in the United States without a doctor's prescription. Androstenedione is banned by many sports organizations outside of baseball including the National Football League (NFL) and the International Olympic Committee (IOC). Despite the fact that McGwire's actions were legal and within the rules of Major League Baseball, many sports observers were dismayed. "In raising his testosterone to reach Maris's record," wrote syndicated columnist Derrick Z. Jackson, "McGwire has lowered the values of his sport. No longer is it the best man who wins. It is the best-enhanced man." (In August 1999, McGwire announced that he had stopped using the substance. He hit sixty-five home runs in the 1999 season.)

McGwire was not the first—or the last—high profile athlete to take so-called performance-enhancing drugs. In 1998 alone several significant drug scandals shook the sports world. Irish swimmer Michelle de Bruin, winner of three gold medals in the 1996 Atlanta Olympics, was banned from swimming competitions after submitting a suspicious urine sample to drug testers. American shotputter Randy Barnes, an Olympic gold medalist, was banned for life from competition for using the same supplement that McGwire used. On the eve of the World Swimming Championships held that year in Australia, Yuan Yuan, a star Chinese swimmer, was arrested at the Sydney airport with thirteen vials of human growth hormone in her possession (enough for the entire team)—a development that seemingly confirmed widespread suspicions that the past success of Chinese women athletes in swimming and other sports was due to drugs. The 1998 Tour de France bicycle race almost collapsed when numerous competitors, including many top teams, were disqualified amid credible allegations that cyclists were systematically using drugs as part of their training regimens.

Taking performance-enhancing drugs, or "doping," has a long history in sport. In 1904, a marathon runner nearly died from a mixture of brandy and strychnine, a poisonous substance that in small quantities acts as a stimulant. Amphetamines replaced strychnine as the stimulant of choice among athletes in the 1930s. In the 1950s, responding to news that Soviet Union weight lifters were being given hormones to increase their strength, physician John Ziegler invented a synthetic substitute—anabolic steroids. Anabolic steroids quickly became popular among athletes, including NFL players, seeking greater muscle growth and strength. From the 1950s through the 1980s, drugs were part of the sports and athletic programs of the Soviet Union and its political allies such as East Germany. Recent investigations have revealed the extent to which many athletes in East Germany and other countries were given steroids and other drugs, sometimes without the athletes' knowledge. The apparent goal for individual countries was to win national glory through victory in sports. Some people believe similar programs currently exist in China. But today, when an Olympic gold medal can mean millions in endorsement dollars, "Doping knows no ideological or geographical boundaries," writes journalist Jason Zengerle, who estimates that more than 30 percent of Olympic athletes use performance drugs.

Some sports events and organizations have banned the use of certain drugs and have implemented programs to test for such substances. The IOC was one of the first organizations to do so. After cyclists believed to be taking amphetamines collapsed and died at the 1960 Olympics and the 1967 Tour de France (not an Olympic event), the IOC established a medical commission and developed a list of banned substances. It began drug testing of contestants at the 1968 Olympic Games. Since then the IOC has continually expanded the list of forbidden substances, which include stimulants, narcotics, steroids, and masking agents (substances meant to hide banned drug use from urine drug tests).

Perhaps the most famous Olympic drug test came after the 100-meter dash at the 1988 Summer Olympics in Seoul. Canadian/Jamaican sprinter Ben Johnson set a world record of 9.79 seconds, but had his gold medal stripped from him when he tested positive for anabolic steroids. Johnson eventually was banned for life from track and field competition. But many believe that Johnson was not the only athlete to abuse drugs. Robert Voy, chief medical officer of the United States Olympic Committee from 1985 to 1989, concluded that "the only thing that separated Johnson from a great number of others who competed in Seoul in a vast variety of sports is simple: He got caught."

In 2000 the IOC helped establish a new World Anti-Doping Agency to coordinate international drug testing efforts in preparation for the 2000 Summer Games in Sydney, Australia. But many have questioned the IOC's commitment against drugs. Some observers have even accused the IOC of concealing positive drug results in past Olympics. The IOC has resisted calls for using blood samples instead of urine samples, for example, or to mandate frequent out-of-competition drug testing. Critics of the IOC argue that it is too wary of alienating corporate sponsors or jeopardizing its ability to market the Olympics if the true extent of athletic drug use were to be revealed. Speaking of the negative public relations fallout from the Ben Johnson incident, health professor and steroids expert Charles Yesalis asserted in a 1999 *Newsweek* article that the IOC "will never let something like that be made public again. . . . Superstars could have drugs oozing out of their eyeballs and the IOC still wouldn't call it." Danish Sports Minister Elsebeth Berner Nielsen stated in 1999 that "the IOC has proved that they don't have the power or the will to take care of the fight against doping." Many critics of the IOC have called for national governments and other international organizations to take a stronger lead in testing and punishing the use of performance drugs.

The effectiveness of testing has been questioned as well. At the 1996 Atlanta Olympics, there were only two confirmed positive drug tests. For some observers, these low numbers confirmed that athletes had become very successful in circumventing drug tests. Some athletes hide and submit false urine samples. Many use drugs as a training aid between competitions, then stop taking them long enough to test "clean" at the Olympics themselves. Some athletes are turning to substances that occur naturally in the human body, making detection of cheating even more difficult if not impossible. These newly developed substances include human growth hormone (hGH) and erythropoietin (EPO), a hormone that increases oxygen flow to red blood cells. The suspected prevalence of drug use among athletes and the increased sophistication in avoiding positive test results has led to some serious examination of the issue of performance-enhancing drugs in sport. "At its root," writes journalist Christopher P. Winner in *USA Today*, "the doping issue boils down to one hard question: Is it worth trying to keep sports pure by tracking down drug cheats when standards vary and more sophisticated methods make the use of performance-enhancing substances easier to conceal?"

Not all sports observers answer that question in the affirmative. Some argue that drug testing is futile as newer substances are invented and developed. Drug testing can be invasive or degrading, and can produce false positive results that unfairly tarnish an athlete's reputation. Drug regulations are also confusing in that many banned substances may be taken, in some cases inadvertently, through common over-the-counter medications. Moreover, some observers such as medical ethicist Norman Fost argue that athletes should have the right to control what goes into their own bodies. Taking certain drugs to improve one's athletic performance, in this view, differs little in principle from the high altitude training, special diets, and grueling exercise regimens that are commonplace in sports, even though many people outside athletic circles would find these actions "unnatural." Fost and others note that people in other professions often take chemical substances (such as the caffeine in coffee) in order to boost their performance in their vocations, and ask why athletes should be treated differently.

Those who believe athletes should be held to a drug-free standard offer several reasons. Some argue that taking drugs is simply a form of cheating that should not be allowed. Others argue that drug use and suspicion of drug use threaten the enjoyment many people receive from watching athletes compete. "One of the biggest problems with sports today," writes tennis and sports writer Christopher Clarey, "is that whenever someone does something remarkable—sets a world record, runs through the pain, steps suddenly from the shadows into the light—it creates as much suspicion as it does sense of wonder."

Concern for the health of athletes is another reason many oppose drugs in sports. Many performance-enhancing drugs pose health risks. Stimulants can cause changes in heart rhythm and increase blood pressure. Anabolic steroids are linked with liver and heart disorders, psychiatric disturbances, and reduced fertility. They also are blamed for masculinizing effects on women. EPO has been blamed for sudden deaths through blood circulatory failure. Extended use of human growth hormone may cause diabetes, arthritis, or cancer.

Those who worry about health risks argue that many athletes do not really have much of a free choice whether or not to be drug free if cheaters win and typically go uncaught and unpunished. Athletes then are confronted with the dilemma of having to take drugs themselves to give themselves a fighting chance at competing. For athletes who train for years to gain a shot at an Olympic medal or other athletic goal, this can be a difficult choice, although surveys of elite athletes suggest that many would find the temptation difficult to overcome.

The issue of drugs in sports affects more than just elite athletes and their fans. Successful athletes are also seen as role models for the young, many argue, and their actions may have the effect of increasing drug abuse among young people. For example, sales of androstenedione have surged more than 1000 percent since McGwire first admitted to using it, according to industry sources—and much of that increase was attributable to purchases by young people. Some experts have argued that steroid use has doubled among high school athletes over the course of the 1990s and estimate that 18 percent of high school athletes use anabolic steroids.

Whether or not the use of performance-enhancing drugs is something that can ever be fully stopped is one of the issues discussed in *At Issue: Drugs and Sports*. The authors discuss drug use among Olympic, professional, high school, and college athletes, the ethics of doping, and what steps can possibly be taken to prevent it.

1

The Use of Performance-Enhancing Drugs Is Common

Michael Bamberger and Don Yaeger

Michael Bamberger and Don Yaeger write for Sports Illustrated, *a popular weekly sports publication.*

The use of performance-enhancing drugs is prevalent in professional and amateur sports. While many people may associate drug use only with football players or athletes from Europe or Asia, drug use has spread to many sports and has become common in the United States. Many athletes will willingly risk future health damage in order to gain a competitive edge. Most pro leagues and sports organizations do little to prevent drug use, and those that do test for drugs find themselves in a losing battle with athletes and trainers who continually devise new drugs and methods of beating drug tests.

A scenario, from a 1995 poll of 198 sprinters, swimmers, powerlifters and other assorted athletes, most of them U.S. Olympians or aspiring Olympians: You are offered a banned performance-enhancing substance, with two guarantees: 1) You will not be caught. 2) You will win. Would you take the substance?

One hundred and ninety-five athletes said yes; three said no.

Scenario II: You are offered a banned performance-enhancing substance that comes with two guarantees: 1) You will not be caught. 2) You will win every competition you enter for the next five years, and then you will die from the side effects of the substance. Would you take it?

More than half the athletes said yes.

It is no secret that performance-enhancing drugs have been used by Olympians for decades, or that athletes will do almost anything to gain a competitive edge. (Chicago physician and author Bob Goldman has conducted the above survey every two years since 1982 and has gotten more or less the same response each time.) What is surprising is that 25 years

Reprinted from Michael Bamberger and Don Yaeger, "Over the Edge," *Sports Illustrated*, April 14, 1997. Reprinted with permission from *Sports Illustrated*.

after the [1972] introduction of supposedly rigorous drug testing of Olympic athletes, the use of banned performance-enhancing substances has apparently become more widespread, and effective, than ever. "There may be some sportsmen who can win gold medals without taking drugs, but there are very few," says Dutch physician Michel Karsten, who claims to have prescribed anabolic steroids to hundreds of world-class athletes from swimming, track and field and the non-Olympic sport of powerlifting over the last 25 years. "If you are especially gifted, you may win once, but from my experience you can't continue to win without drugs. The field is just too filled with drug users."

Common in many sports

The word steroids calls to mind 325-pound NFL linemen who not so many years ago weighed 250 pounds, or weightlifters with trapezius muscles that ascend like mountains from their shoulders to their ears, or sprinters with quadriceps like steel cables. But the use of steroids—and other, more exotic substances, such as human growth hormone (hGH)—has spread to almost every sport, from major league baseball to college basketball to high school football. It is the dirty and universal secret of sports, amateur and pro, as the millennium draws near.

Though what follows focuses in considerable detail on Olympic sports, circumstantial evidence of performance-enhancing drug use from a wide variety of sports, pro and amateur, abounds. Even casual fans notice that NBA players sport biceps that a Kevin McHale or even a Moses Malone never dreamed of; that Ivy League colleges field football teams with linemen bigger than All-Pro linemen were a few years ago; and that it's no longer remarkable for veteran big league baseball players to show up at spring training having put on 20 pounds of solid muscle since the end of the previous season.

Most pro leagues don't test for performance-enhancing drugs. And those athletic governing bodies that do, strike fear in the hearts of few athletes. The International Olympic Committee (IOC) sanctioned exactly two positive drug tests at last summer's [1996] Atlanta Games out of a pool of 11,000 athletes, 2,000 of whom were tested for banned substances. No medals were forfeited. From those numbers—down from five positives at the 1992 Olympics in Barcelona and the all-time high of 12 positives at the '84 Games in Los Angeles—you might assume that the '96 Olympics were the cleanest since the beginning of full-scale drug testing at the '72 Games. Don't kid yourself.

> *Circumstantial evidence of performance-enhancing drug use from a wide variety of sports . . . abounds.*

Dozens of athletes, coaches, administrators and steroid traffickers interviewed by *Sports Illustrated* (*SI*) say that the Atlanta Olympics, like other Games of the last half century, was a carnival of sub-rosa experiments in the use of performance-enhancing drugs. And few of those interviewed were surprised that only two users were caught. "Athletes are a walking laboratory, and the Olympics have become a proving ground for scientists, chemists and unethical doctors," says Dr. Robert Voy, the director of drug testing for the U.S. Olympic Committee (USOC) at the 1984 and '88 Games. "The testers know that the [drug] gurus are smarter than they are. They know how to get in under the radar."

No less an authority than Dr. Donald Catlin, director of the IOC-accredited drug-testing lab at UCLA, while noting that "I don't think everyone in Atlanta was doped," makes a telling admission: "The sophisticated athlete who wants to take drugs has switched to things we can't test for."

The IOC itself has scheduled a summit to address the state of drug testing in Lausanne, Switzerland, on April 22–23 [1997]. Since the Olympics, it has pointed to the testing results in Atlanta more than once as evidence that testing discourages drug use. But critics describe the IOC's testing program as crippled by bureaucracy and politics, tolerance for the use of banned substances and flawed testing methods. The $2.5 million drug-testing effort in Atlanta was, in fact, almost comically ineffective. To augment testing done with a gas chromatograph mass spectrometer (the device that turned up the two positives), the IOC brought in a vaunted new piece of equipment, the high-resolution mass spectrometer (HRMS), that would supposedly be able to catch athletes who had used steroids in the previous two or three months. During the Games the HRMS revealed what appeared to be five positive tests for anabolic steroids. But the IOC threw the results out. Olympic officials, fearful of expensive lawsuits—many an athlete who has tested positive for steroids has sued an athletic federation, the IOC, a lab or a meet sponsor—decided that the positive tests might not stand up in court because the mass spectrometer was still relatively untested.

> *There's a saying that to be a great athlete today you need a great coach, a great chemist and a great lawyer.*

Even if the IOC's equipment were both proven and technologically cutting-edge, eliminating drug use from Olympic sports would be no small challenge. The users range from weightlifters and shot-putters and bobsledders to swimmers and marathoners and gymnasts. (While male gymnasts might typically turn to steroids to get stronger, some female gymnasts are said to intentionally retard their growth by taking so-called brake drugs, such as cyproterone acetate, a substance sometimes used to reduce the sex drive in hyperlibidinous men.) Says Kees Kooman, the editor of the Dutch edition of *Runner's World* magazine, "All athletes someday have to choose: Do I want to compete at a world-class level and take drugs, or do I want to compete at a club level and be clean?"

Over the years athletes from the former Eastern-bloc countries, the Netherlands and China have been known as heavy users of performance-enhancing drugs, but American Olympians, at least in the eyes of the U.S. public, never have been so stigmatized. That is a misperception. "I've had American athletes tell me they were doing performance-enhancing drugs," says Voy. "Most of these athletes didn't really want to do drugs.

But they would come to me and say, 'Unless you stop the drug abuse in sport, I have to do drugs. I'm not going to spend the next two years training—away from my family, missing my college education—to be an Olympian and then be cheated out of a medal by some guy from Europe or Asia who is on drugs.'"

"I would say nearly every top-level athlete is on something," says Michael Mooney, a California bodybuilder and authority on steroids who used to help athletes with questions on how to use the drugs most effectively and now designs steroid regimens for AIDS doctors to prescribe to their patients. "What bothers me are the hypocrites, the athletes I've talked to who I later read are talking about how bad steroids are. The number of these supposed steroid-free athletes—very well-known athletes—who have contacted me about how to pass [drug] tests in just the last year blows my mind."

In 1993 the head of the IOC's medical commission, Prince Alexandre de Merode of Belgium, told a British newspaper that he believed that as many as 10% of all Olympic athletes were regular users of performance-enhancing drugs. At the time, that statement made headlines. Now the 10% estimate seems hopelessly naive. In a rambling interview with *SI*, De Merode said, "I am not unhappy about the situation. More and more, high-level athletes have to be treated like normal workers. We have to be able to face the courts. People don't realize that our power is very weak. We have power only at the Olympic Games. The federations and national governing bodies have . . . more power. Everybody is doing it. Nobody is taking note that an actor, a singer, a politician or a truck driver is taking drugs. They don't have tests. We have tests. We have made a lot of progress."

Avoiding detection

Drug insiders see it differently. According to those interviewed by *SI*, three distinct classes of top-level athletes have emerged in many Olympic sports. One is a small group of athletes who are not using any banned performance enhancers. The second is a large, burgeoning group whose drug use goes undetected; these athletes either take drugs that aren't tested for, use tested-for drugs in amounts below the generous levels permitted by the IOC or take substances that mask the presence of the drugs in their system at testing time. The third group comprises the smattering of athletes who use banned performance enhancers and are actually caught. To be caught is not easy; it only happens, says Emil Vrijman, director of the Netherlands' doping control center, when an athlete is either incredibly sloppy, incredibly stupid or both.

Of course, avoiding detection does require an effort. The days of an athlete's simply turning in a bottle of somebody else's urine are over. As degrading as it may sound, an official is now required to watch the athlete urinate. Even that's not foolproof: Cases have been reported of an athlete urinating before an event, inserting a catheter up his or her urethra and using the equivalent of a turkey baster to squeeze someone else's urine into his or her bladder.

Of course, an athlete who refines his use of banned performance enhancers need not worry about giving a urine sample. If an athlete stops taking water-based steroids—the most common kind—within two weeks, there is, typically, no detectable drug left in his urine. And that's being cautious. Says Ben Johnson, the Canadian sprinter who was stripped of his gold medal in the 100 meters after testing positive for anabolic steroids at the 1988 Olympics, "There are about six dozen drugs on the market, as far as I know, and some, like water-based testosterone, leave the system in a day," an assertion confirmed by several experts on steroids and other performance-enhancing substances. Even with the most commonly used water-based steroids, the two-week period can be shortened. "Let's say I have a deal with a lab under which I can send your urine to test your [steroid] levels," says Voy, assuming the role of an illicit-drug adviser. "Then I just play around. I adjust the doses. I know exactly when to get you off to fall below the [drug-testing] radar. If I can get you off nine days before your event, we've got it made, because chances are you're not going to lose any of your [strength and endurance] gains in that period. It's simple biochemistry."

"I know athletes who take their urine to a women's health center in West Hollywood," says California-based steroid expert Jim Brockman, a self-trained biochemist and trainer whom athletes have contacted about steroid use and how to hide it. "The lab is important. You have to constantly monitor your usage."

Drug gurus

But what about the random, out-of-competition testing conducted by some sports federations, including FINA, swimming's world governing body? Doesn't that scare athletes?

Not much. There's a saying that to be a great athlete today you need a great coach, a great chemist and a great lawyer. The so-called chemists—who in fact are just as likely to be trainers, doctors or simply self-taught drug experts—are known in the athletic community as gurus. They specialize in buying illicit performance-boosting substances and creating programs that will give a client maximum benefit from those substances while minimizing his chances of getting caught. "No athlete I've ever helped has tested positive, and I've helped hundreds," says a Dutch doctor who has been a guru. The athletes he has helped, the guru-doctor says, come from "every sport you can imagine."

Gurus often buy or create so-called designer steroids for athletes who can afford the price of a program (as much as $3,000 a month). These drugs are steroids that have been chemically altered to tailor them to an athlete's needs and render them more difficult for testers to identify. Each type of steroid has a unique signature that shows up in the urine of a user. Because drug testers look only for the signatures of commercially available steroids, a steroid whose signature has been changed will be much more difficult to detect. For an athlete using that altered steroid, passing a drug test becomes a breeze.

Even an athlete with little money can have his steroids doctored. Despite the many polysyllabic terms bandied about in the steroid culture, the chemical components of steroids are so simple to alter that virtually any graduate student in chemistry has the ability to do it. *SI* took one guru's steroid-altering instructions to a third-year college chemistry student, who in the course of two days made the resultant designer drug. An independent testing lab, which analyzed the altered drug, said that its testers would be unable to find any identifiable trace of steroids in the urine of any person who had taken the designer drug.

Drug gurus are so easily found that an *SI* writer tracked down three of them—one in Houston, another in Kingston, Jamaica, and a third in Denver—by making a half-dozen telephone calls over the course of a week. The guru in Houston, a chemist who once worked for a pharmaceutical company, did not want the writer to visit him. "There are too many people here you'd recognize," he said.

To procure drugs, American gurus go to local doctors, to pharmacies in Tijuana, to dealers hanging out at bodybuilding gyms all over the U.S., to track and field meets in Europe.

The gurus do all their business in cash; the cash is provided by the athletes. A guru who is a doctor risks losing his license by providing an athlete with any performance-enhancing substance, such as an anabolic steroid, that by law can only be prescribed for bona fide medical needs. But the doctor has incentives. A kilogram of pure testosterone wholesales for $500 through medical channels. It can be mixed with calcium, made into tablets and produce about $100,000 in illicit steroid sales, according to the U.S. Drug Enforcement Administration. (An athlete caught possessing steroids without a prescription could likewise face a felony rap, but that's just another risk many athletes are more than willing to take.)

After the guru buys and perhaps alters a drug, his next job is to make sure it is administered properly—that is, in a way that will enhance performance without being detected. The trick is for the athlete to receive just the right dosage at just the right time.

The guru might tell a sprinter, "You should take 40 milligrams of Winstrol [a steroid] three times a week for eight weeks, then take nothing for eight weeks, then resume your schedule for six weeks until three weeks before your competition." One of the guru's most important roles is to hold the athlete back; athletes, like junkies or alcoholics, often take the view that if a little is good, more is better.

Popular substances

Actually, for sprinters and other strength athletes, the most popular banned substance today is human growth hormone, not steroids. (Some athletes jokingly referred to the Atlanta Olympics as the Growth Hormone Games.) Growth hormone is used primarily by pediatricians to treat dwarfism, but it also helps an athlete's muscles recover speedily from intense workouts and thereby enables him or her to train harder and more often. Urine tests don't detect hGH, which is one reason so many athletes are taking injections of it despite the $1,500-a-month cost.

While growth hormone is popular among strength athletes, competitors who rely on endurance—long-distance runners, cross-country skiers, distance swimmers and the like—prefer a genetically engineered version of erythropoietin, or EPO, a natural hormone that is effective in the treatment of kidney disease, anemia and other disorders. It stimulates the formation of red blood cells, which carry oxygen to the muscles, thus fostering greater endurance for athletes. Urine testing cannot detect EPO use. And though more than two dozen deaths have been attributed to

EPO—including the deaths of five Dutch cyclists in 1987, the year the drug was introduced in Europe—its popularity among athletes persists. "You have guys who will go to the funeral of a friend who died from this stuff, come home and inject it again," says an Olympic distance runner from Europe who uses EPO himself. There is an ongoing effort to find urine tests for both EPO and hGH, so far to no avail.

The frustration of drug-testers might be reduced with one bold move: The IOC could require the testing of athletes' blood. Blood testing can detect signs of illicit usage of both hGH and EPO. Since March [1997] the UCI, cycling's worldwide governing body, responding to riders' requests, has been testing the blood of professional road racers for signs of EPO. Four cyclists found to have thickened blood have been forced to sit out races as a "health precaution."

Catlin maintains that blood testing is not yet reliable enough to be used at the Olympics. Other testing experts disagree but see it as impractical. "Blood testing is invasive," says Goldman, whose book, *Death in the Locker Room,* last updated in 1995, details the dangers of steroid use and abuse. "Blood's too much of a pain. Blood spoils. Tubes break. It can clot if you don't keep it cool when shipping. You're sticking holes in athletes, and some people have religious problems with that. People pass out. But blood testing would be more accurate. There's no doubt about that."

So why no official push for blood testing? Says Voy, "It's very difficult for sport organizations that depend on sponsorship money" to have their athletes caught taking performance enhancers. "The IOC fears exposing the high levels of drug use. It turns off the public. The IOC is very nervous about testing."

Testing in the Olympics

Voy quit his Olympic position in 1989 because, he says, neither the IOC nor the USOC was committed to eliminating the use of illicit performance enhancers. Exposing star athletes would create enough publicity to send sponsors packing, and it might also disillusion a sports-watching public that assumes that the overwhelming majority of Olympic athletes are clean.

Once scientists determine that the drug test of an Olympic athlete is positive, two separate IOC committees must accept the results. The committees meet in private and have been accused of putting the interests of a particular sport or a particular country ahead of the drug-testing rules. Ontario Supreme Court judge Charles Dubin, who as head of the 1989 Canadian government inquiry into drug use in sports heard months of testimony, concluded that the IOC had by omission covered up more drug use than it had uncovered. "The general public has long been led to assume that if only one athlete tested positive, the others were not also using drugs," wrote Dubin in his report. "We know now, as the IOC . . . has known for many years, that this assumption is false."

Nor is the testing itself as stringent as Olympic testers would have the public believe. The IOC tolerates startlingly high levels of testosterone in both male and female athletes. Olympic testing guidelines established 15 years ago by the late German biochemist Manfred Donike, who was the head of the IOC's doping subcommittee from 1980 until his death in

1995, measure an athlete's testosterone level as a ratio between the testosterone and the epitestosterone (a natural hormone with no known physiological benefit) found in his or her urine. Virtually all men have a testosterone/epitestosterone (t/e) ratio of 1.3 to 1 or lower. A small fraction of men, far fewer than 10 in 1,000, have a t/e ratio of more than 5 to 1. To cover these people and to avoid lawsuits, Donike pegged the maximum acceptable ratio in Olympic athletes at 6 to 1. Thus, a male athlete with a natural t/e ratio of 1 to 1 can artificially increase his ratio to 6 to 1 and still have legal readings. A man with a natural 1-to-1 ratio could take 200 milligrams of testosterone three times a week and remain below 6 to 1. Sports scientists say that a run-of-the-mill male athlete with a 1-to-1 t/e ratio who raised his ratio to 6 to 1 by injecting testosterone, in conjunction with hGH, could improve his athletic performance by as much as 10% to 20%. That's a huge advantage in, say, a 100-meter sprint, in which a few hundredths of a second can separate first place from fourth, or in a throwing event, in which six feet can separate a gold medalist from an also-ran.

Some athletes jokingly referred to the Atlanta Olympics as the Growth Hormone Games.

Donike also established 6 to 1 as the legal ratio for women, even though it is almost unheard of for a woman to have a ratio greater than 2.5 to 1.

A woman who boosted her ratio to 6 to 1 would see even more dramatic improvements in performance than a man who did so. "Women require a lot less anabolic stimulation than men do in order to build up their strength and endurance," says Voy. "It's sometimes pretty hard to stimulate a lot of males with anabolic steroids because a lot of their androgen receptor sites [male-hormone receptors found in almost every muscle in the body] for the anabolic steroids have been closed down because of maturity. But in a woman those receptor sites are always open, so just a little tweak here and you can get great gains."

Donike's guidelines have had the unintended effect of encouraging female athletes to take more powerful muscle-building substances. Before Donike established the 6-to-1 t/e ratio, says Mooney, "women preferred synthetically produced steroids over straight testosterone because the synthetics had fewer male side effects. Since then, it's been easier to get by the tests with pure testosterone, so that's what they're using." He adds, "You start feeding a woman testosterone, essentially you're turning her physiology into a man."

That and other risks from banned performance-enhancing substances are well-documented. Steroids can cause heart disease, liver cancer and impotence. The hormone of the moment, hGH, can cause disfigurement by encouraging growth not only of muscles but also of bones, especially in the feet, hands and face. Some hGH users develop jutting foreheads, prominent cheekbones and an elongated jaw. (In Olympic circles an athlete with a pronounced chin is sometimes said to have GH jaw.) According to Walter Jekot, a Los Angeles pediatrician doing five years in North Las Vegas Federal Prison following his 1992 conviction for trafficking in steroids, a track athlete had to undergo a skin graft in the late 1980s because doses of hGH had caused the bones to practically push through the skin, and the athlete could no longer fully open his hands.

None of that has stopped athletes from using performance-boosting drugs. They are skeptical not only of the proposition that testing will catch them but also of the proposition that it will catch their competition. "We've lost the trust of the athlete," says Vrijman, the Netherlands' testing official. Ironically, the IOC catalog of 200 banned substances has come to serve as a shopping list. "The best advertisement for athletes to find drugs is to put them on the banned list," says Vrijman. The logic is impeccable: "That tells the athlete that this drug improves performance, or we wouldn't ban it."

And every year there is new stuff to try. One performance-boosting substance growing in popularity is Insulin Growth Factor-1. Since it is naturally produced by the body, the presence of IGF-1 in a urine sample can be explained away easily. Insulin pulls nutrients into muscle tissue, thus promoting muscle growth.

In Atlanta traces of a drug relatively new to testers appeared in the urine samples of athletes from Russia and other Eastern European countries. The stimulant was ultimately identified as bromantan, and its use by athletes was so new—although it had been used by the Russian military to keep troops alert and to adapt quickly to extreme heat and cold—it was not yet on the banned list. The drug's benefits were not fully understood, nor its dangers. That hardly mattered. When the word that bromantan had the potential to improve performances got around, the drug did too.

A great silence enshrouds the world of covert drug use. What athlete wants to confess to a practice that would taint the authenticity of his performance—and to a felony to boot? Retired athletes too have no incentive to tell a truth that would bring shame to their careers. A British bobsledder, Mark Tout, failed a drug test in 1996 and openly discussed his steroid use. That inspired exactly no one else to come forward.

A great silence enshrouds the whole world of covert drug use.

The continuing pervasiveness of drugs in the Olympics and other sports competitions has even spawned a small but vocal movement that promotes legalizing the use of anabolic steroids and other banned substances. One who has articulated this argument is Dr. Norman Fost, a visiting professor of bioethics at Princeton, who says in lectures and writings that steroids are not appreciably different from certain legal foods and drugs that enhance performance and that the health risks of steroids have been seriously exaggerated. "The widespread use of anabolic steroids by athletes is upsetting to many people, but it is not clear why," Fost began a 1983 piece published by *The New York Times*. "The objection that steroids provide an 'unnatural' assist to performance is inchoate. Many of the means and ends which athletes use and seek are unnatural. From Nautilus machines to . . . Gatorade, their lives are filled with drugs and devices whose aim is to maximize performance."

That's nuts, says Catlin. If drugs were permitted, he says, "then we would just have a race among pharmacologists to find better and stronger drugs. Now at least they [athletes] have to worry about being detected."

Clearly, that race is already on, and drug testing is serving as no deterrent. "People like to think that things are better since Ben Johnson," says Dutch track coach Henk Kraayenhof, who has trained world-class runners for 20 years. "I argue the opposite. If anything, Ben Johnson's getting caught promoted drug use.

"He won."

2

Steroid Use Is a Growing Problem Among American High School Athletes

Gary Mihoces

Gary Mihoces is a reporter for the newspaper USA Today.

The number of American middle and high school students abusing steroids is growing. Many teens use these drugs, which are related to male sex hormones, to improve athletic performance or personal appearance. However, these substances are legal only by prescription and carry significant health risks.

We're used to football players or Olympians getting caught using steroids now and again.

This might shock you: A national survey shows a rise in steroid use by eighth- and 10th-grade boys. Though use was lower among girls, it rose, too. It was higher among girls in eighth grade than 12th grade.

"I'm alarmed, not only because of each individual, but the fact that it's growing," says Don Herrmann, chairman of the sports medicine committee for the National Federation of State High School Associations.

"Where is that all going to stop? How much faster is it going to grow?"

The National Institute on Drug Abuse (NIDA) has a new campaign to prevent use of steroids by young people—whether athletes looking for better performance or non-athletes lured by images of the body beautiful.

The campaign includes a new NIDA Web site: www.steroidabuse.org.

There is no temptation to use steroids for Joey Hess and Chris Lewis, 15-year-old athletes at Southport High in Indianapolis.

"I've heard a lot of dangers. Loss of hair, all that stuff," says Hess, who plays football and baseball.

"I'd like to get big on my own, do something I could be proud of," says Lewis, a basketball player.

But they say they wonder when they hear about some junior high kid bench-pressing 300 pounds.

The 1999 Monitoring the Future study surveyed 45,000 students in the eighth, 10th and 12th grades at 433 schools. About one in 40 boys in eighth and 10th grade said they had used steroids the previous year. Among girls, it remained less than one per 100, but it rose in all three grades.

Penn State professor Charles Yesalis estimates 175,000 teenage girls and 375,000 teenage boys in the USA have used steroids at one time or another.

You might know lots of teenagers and not suspect any of steroid use.

"I've never heard of it, and I certainly wouldn't approve of it," says Cindy Knecht, a parent from Johnstown, Ohio.

Her daughter, Caroline, 13, an eighth-grader, plays softball and volleyball. She, too, is surprised by the survey: "Nobody I know."

Her friend, Stephanie Shoaf, 14, plays basketball and softball. She's only heard about steroids on the news, "like the stuff football players take to make them stronger."

Yesalis says use can be hidden from friends and families.

"The secrecy surrounding steroids is dramatically greater than the use of other so-called street drugs," he says. He says some steroid use might have a parental OK: "I get a couple of calls a year asking me to kind of give my blessing to getting their kids on steroids."

Illegal drugs

Steroids are laboratory-made versions of the human hormone testosterone, which aids growth of muscles, bones and skin. Testosterone is primarily a male hormone. Females produce trace amounts.

Steroids may be legally prescribed by doctors for some medical uses. Steroids for muscle-building are obtained illegally. They are produced overseas or in clandestine laboratories in the USA.

For all of the health risks, part of the dilemma is research shows steroids do work when it comes to building muscles and power.

"These things, in my judgment, work better than most scientists believe," Yesalis says. "The athletes figured out how well these work long before scientists."

The muscle-building effects tend to be more quickly apparent in adolescents and females.

Numerous side effects [of steroids] can include breast enlargement for males, growth of facial hair for females and severe acne for both.

"When the receptor sites in their bodies, which don't have much testosterone in them, suddenly are presented with a lot of testosterone, they get activated," says Gary Wadler of the New York University School of Medicine. "They'll get more muscular, more defined. They'll lose some fat, increase their lean body mass, get stronger."

But the numerous side effects can include breast enlargement for males, growth of facial hair for females and severe acne for both.

Among adolescents, there can be stunted skeletal growth, NIDA says.

While there are no studies of long-term steroid use, researchers suspect it can heighten the risk of liver cancer, heart attack and stroke.

All that doesn't discourage some.

"Surveys that indicate what people are willing to do in order to win frighten me," says Steve Roush, assistant executive director of USA Swimming. "There is a population out there that will go above and beyond what is healthy and ethical."

Studies show steroid use is more prevalent in sports such as football and the weight events in track.

"But it's been shown to be in all sports," Yesalis says.

Steroids are taken in tablet form or by injection, usually in cycles over several weeks. They are banned by sports governing bodies and leagues around the world.

Illegal steroids typically are sold in gyms and health clubs and by mail. Now, the Internet is another avenue. "There are numerous sites selling products, selling 'real' anabolic steroids, which is not to say all of it is real stuff," Yesalis says.

He says an eight-week cycle of steroids can cost anywhere from a couple of hundred dollars to a couple of thousand, depending on dose, type and availability.

Two hundred dollars sounds expensive for high school students. But remember, some pay almost that much for sneakers.

Increase baffling

Why the big jump among young boys?

"I don't think anybody knows," says Alan Leshner, director of the National Institute on Drug Abuse. . . .

"Some people are going to imply that it has to do with one or more athletes. . . . I'm not sure that's fair."

Lloyd Johnston is the principal investigator for the Monitoring the Future study by the University of Michigan's Institute for Social Research.

He has a theory that he describes as "pure conjecture" because the students surveyed weren't asked about it: "This was a broad change, one we saw all over the country. . . . And about the only thing you can think of in that historical period was the event of Mark McGwire's use of andro becoming public knowledge—not that he intended for that to happen."

During the 1998 season, while McGwire was breaking baseball's home run record, the public was introduced to androstenedione, aka andro.

After a reporter spotted a bottle of it in his locker, McGwire acknowledged using andro—which is sold over the counter without prescription. It's not regulated by the U.S. Food and Drug Administration because it is classified as a dietary supplement, not a drug.

McGwire said last season that he had stopped using andro, even though it's not banned by baseball. "I don't like the way it was portrayed that I was the endorser of the product," he said.

"I discourage young children from taking it."

Andro a steroid?

The Monitoring the Future study did not ask students whether they used andro. Johnston acknowledges that some of those who said they used steroids might have been referring to andro.

Yesalis on andro: "These are only supplements by a legal loophole."

Wadler says the legal status of andro sends a conflicting message: "Anabolic steroids are classified as controlled substances. Steroid precursors like androstenedione have been deregulated by Congress. You can't have it both ways."

But some young people already are going beyond andro to steroids.

In response, some high schools test for steroids. But it is costly, as much as $125 a student, and schools that test are rare.

Linn Goldberg of Oregon Health Sciences University has just published a report on an alternative method. His study reports steroid use was reduced among high school football players in Oregon through a program that used students to teach students about the health hazards of steroids.

"It's not, 'Just Say No.' A negative message won't work," Goldberg says. "I think a reasonable alternative with a positive message will work."

3

State-Sponsored Drug Use Has Tarnished the Olympic Games

Richard Panek

Richard Panek writes for the periodical Women's Sports & Fitness.

The issue of drugs in sports has special poignancy for members of the U.S. women's swim team who competed in the 1976 Summer Olympics. Heavily favored to win, they were instead badly beaten by the East Germans, and many swimmers were castigated for losing and for voicing suspicions of drug use among the victors. But developments after the fall of the Berlin Wall in 1989 have revealed the extent to which the country of East Germany during the 1970s and 1980s engaged in a systematic program of drugging athletes with the intent of winning medals at the Olympic Games. Efforts to gain appropriate official recognition for the American swimmers have been rebuffed. Widespread suspicions of drug use persist among Olympic athletes.

They weren't the favorites. In 1976, in international competition, second best was still a new position for U.S. women swimmers to find themselves in, but there they were: As they lined up for their first event in the Montreal Summer Olympics, the 400-meter medley relay, Shirley Babashoff, Camille Wright, Lauri Siering and Linda Jezek couldn't necessarily anticipate a victory. Four years earlier, in Munich, America's women swimmers had won gold medals in six individual events and two relays; the East Germans, none. Since then, however, the East Germans had begun breaking world records in swimming with astonishing frequency. They were big, strong and fast—that unlikely but, in swimming, most desirable combination of physical traits. More to the point, the East Germans were now bigger, stronger and faster on average than the U.S. women. Which is not to say that the Americans didn't think they could win. If each swimmer reached inside and somehow did better than her previous personal best, then maybe, just maybe, the four young members of the

Reprinted from Richard Panek, "Tarnished Gold," *Women's Sports & Fitness*, May/June 1999. Reprinted with permission from the author.

1976 U.S. women's Olympic swim team would bring home the gold.

It wasn't even close.

Four minutes, seven and 95/100 seconds after the crack of the starter's pistol, the last woman on the East German relay team touched the tile that marked the finish of the race. The last of the U.S. swimmers reached the wall 6.6 seconds later—in racing terms, a lifetime. Canada followed, and then the other teams in rapid succession, as you might expect from a race at the highest level of competition. What you wouldn't expect was the vast disparity between the winners and everyone else in the world. As *The New York Times* succinctly summarized the outcome the following day, the American swimmers "seemed to be in another race."

In a way, they were, though some say they didn't realize it at the time. "I was 16 years old," says Linda Wittwer (then Jezek). "I thought [the people] running things knew what they were doing, so that if the East Germans were cheating, it would come up."

Others, however, knew. "It was obvious!" says Lauri Siering, another swimmer on the 400-meter medley relay. "It was pretty well accepted among the swimmers that, yes, they were using steroids."

In the summer of 1998, for the first time, trainers and doctors admitted in a German court of law that throughout the '70s and '80s the East German government routinely and methodically administered illegal performance-enhancing drugs to athletes, including unwitting minors, as part of a formal program not only to win Olympic recognition but to prove the superiority of the socialist system.

In a way, these confessions and convictions only proved what international athletic observers had long assumed to be true. As USA Swimming outside counsel Richard R. Young puts it, "The sun rises in the east and sets in the west, and East Germany was drugging the bejesus out of its athletes." Still, these conclusions were now official—the Olympic equivalent of getting O.J. to say "I did it"—and further support for the growing popular impression that the Olympic rings had come unhinged.

The Olympics, of course, have never been free of politics: Hitler staged the 1936 Berlin Games as a pageant of Aryan supremacy, and terrorists attacked Israeli athletes at the 1972 Munich Games. The Salt Lake City site selection scandal [involving alleged bribes to those responsible for choosing Olympic sites] is merely an example of municipal graft writ large. What Cold War politics wrought in 1976, however, was corruption from within—an agenda to alter the actual competitions and influence their outcomes.

Revisiting the 1976 Olympics

Now, thanks to the trials, investigators could match names of doctors and coaches to names of East German athletes; athletes to events; events, maybe, to medals. In the fall of 1998, the U.S. Olympic Committee (USOC) selected one such event, the 400-meter medley relay, and petitioned the International Olympic Committee (IOC) to amend the record books and award a new set of medals to the runners-up. Suddenly athletes whose bad luck it was to come of age at the same time as juiced-up East Germans found themselves revisiting the Games of their youth and the girls they were then, and wondering what's become of them both.

Camille Wright-Thompson (then Wright), a third member of the 400-meter medley relay, remembers the first time she got a look at the East German swimmers at a meet in Concord, California in 1975. She recalls walking into the pool area and seeing some swimmers standing against the wall with their backs to her. Wow, those are big guys, she thought, and then she noticed something: shoulder straps.

"'These are the girls!'" she remembers telling another American. "'They're not the men—these are the girls we've got to swim against!' That blew us away." Other swimmers recall walking into the locker room, hearing those deep voices and reflexively thinking, Wrong room! The differences were impossible to ignore. Before one race, Wright-Thompson says, she was trying to block out the swimmers standing on either side of her. Then, from the next lane, she heard a cough. A deep cough. A man's cough. Wright-Thompson couldn't help herself. She looked. "And I thought, Oh, gosh—I wasn't supposed to do that!"

To say that the East Germans had undergone a startling metamorphosis since the previous Olympics would be an understatement. In 1972, the only East German swimmer of note was Kornelia Ender, then 13, who won three medals, all silver. Yet within a year East German women swimmers were breaking world records with matter-of-fact regularity, winning 10 of 14 events at the 1973 Belgrade world championships. By the 1976 Games, East Germany's women held a staggering 12 of 13 world records.

Officially, the East Germans attributed their swimmers' success to a superior regimen that devoted at least a quarter of training time to weight lifting. Promising athletes were identified at an early age, removed from the care of their parents and cocooned in special facilities, approximately 20 clubs where 12,000 athletes ate, slept, attended classes and trained. Years later they would emerge, butterflies of bodybuilding, symbols of the socialist work ethic triumphant.

Even so, their rivals privately doubted that such dramatic changes, either competitively or physiologically, were possible without pharmaceutical help—specifically, steroids. Among themselves, swimmers began to refer to the East Germans as "bionic women." U.S. athletes speculated, too, but they couldn't afford to let the East Germans distract them. "The coaches said, 'Yeah, it's obvious they're doing that, but you guys still have a job to do,'" says Siering. Adds Wright-Thompson, "If you're thinking about them too much, you're a sure loser."

As the week in Montreal wore on, it became more of a struggle for the Americans to pretend not to notice what seemed, at least to some of them, painfully unfair. On the second day of competition, Kim Peyton and Karen Moe Thornton set American records in the 100-meter freestyle and the 200-meter butterfly. Neither time was good enough even for a bronze. The East Germans Kornelia Ender and Andrea Pollack set a world record and an Olympic record, respectively, in the same events. The following day, the premier American woman swimmer, Shirley Babashoff, beat the world record in the 400-meter freestyle . . . but so did the East German Petra Thümer, who reached the tile one and a half feet ahead of Babashoff. After the race, Thümer approached Babashoff, who turned her back.

The snub was a spectacular breach of Olympic etiquette but not inconsistent with Babashoff's natural intensity. "Shirley's a nice person," her coach explained, "but her competitiveness can make her mean."

More to the point, the gesture reflected her mounting frustration, resentment and anger. For Babashoff, 1976 was going to be her year. She had won one gold and two silvers at the Munich Games, the USOC had named her Sportswoman of the Year in 1974, and at the 1976 Olympic trials, she'd broken the world record in the 800-meter freestyle. Now she was 19 and at the height of her formidable powers. She had entered the Games as "the next Mark Spitz," but suddenly she found herself in danger of becoming a symbol of athletic misfortune, a regrettable original: the first Shirley Babashoff.

Publicly, she strained to be diplomatic. As the top American swimmer, she was the unofficial spokeswoman the press turned to for answers about the disappointing U.S. performance. "I feel great," she said, after her second-place finish in the 400-meter freestyle. What about the East Germans—are they that good? "We're all swimming well." And what about U.S. hopes for a gold? "We're trying."

The day after she lost to Thümer, Babashoff visited her mother at a nearby hotel, collapsed on her shoulder and sobbed. The East Germans were cheating her out of not only her last chance at Olympic glory but her rightful place in sports history. When she turned her back, she was sending a message she didn't dare put into words, at least not yet.

By the end of the week, East Germany had won golds in 11 of 13 events, in the process setting eight world records. Babashoff took the unprecedented step of sitting out the 400-meter individual medley to save herself for the final two events. The strategy worked. She came in second in the 800-meter freestyle—her fourth silver—and led the United States to its only gold, in the 400-meter freestyle relay. "Here we were, awesome," recalls Siering, "and they just kicked butt."

At first, some U.S. swimmers figured they wouldn't need to address East German drug use directly. The press seemed ready to do it for them. "Among other things whispered about East German athletes," *Sports Illustrated* had reported, "is that they are beefed up, especially the women, by anabolic steroids." At the Summer Games, one journalist baited East German coach Rolf Gläser about the deep voices of the women on his team. "We're here to swim, not to sing," Gläser snapped back, a response that achieved widespread notoriety.

Then there were the new, official antidrug measures. Even when drug tests came back negative, rivals figured that the East Germans had developed strategies for escaping detection, not that they were clean. "The East Germans tested fine," says Wendy Boglioli, who won a bronze medal for the United States in the 100-meter butterfly and a gold in the 400-meter freestyle relay, "but we knew they were on something."

The aftermath

After the Olympics, Boglioli told the press that she "suspected the East Germans of using steroids to build strong women athletes." What was apparent to Boglioli and her fellow athletes, however, didn't seem so obvious to everyone else. In the aftermath of the accusations, an angry consensus quickly formed on the nation's op-ed pages: The Americans were suffering from "sour grapes," read a letter to *The New York Times*. Their remarks "reek of jealousy, cattiness and cruelty," said another letter, and a third suggested, "Possibly, our women swimmers should look beyond the count of their medals to the ideal of the spirit of competition and friendship that these Games are to espouse."

What ideal? For Boglioli, the memories didn't square with the official Olympic philosophy. "The idea of the Games is to get young people together and create understanding, but there was none of this," she lamented in a speech soon after the Games. "Some of the countries herded their athletes to and from events and I think locked them in dorms when they weren't competing or practicing. We never saw them."

The East German government routinely and methodically administered illegal performance-enhancing drugs to athletes, including unwitting minors.

For Boglioli and the other athletes who had publicly speculated about East German drug use, the worst was still to come: death threats. For a year and a half after Montreal, Boglioli asked the FBI to check her mail and tap her phone.

Meanwhile, the East Germans went home as heroes who had shown the world that a nation of 17 million could sweep the Olympics, amassing 90 medals in all—second only to the U.S.S.R. and ahead of the United States. "This proves the success of our socialist system and training methods," proclaimed Manfred Ewald, president of the country's Olympic committee. Kornelia Ender, then 17, who led East Germany with four golds (including, incredibly, individual golds only 27 minutes apart, in the 100-meter butterfly and the 200-meter freestyle), attributed her nation's success to "the generous encouragement and aid given the athletes by the party, the working class and the government."

"It just infuriated me," Boglioli says, and clearly it still does. "For people to say we got beat because they were better than us? No. I was the best. Camille: the best. Shirley: the best."

And yet?

"And yet"—she shrugs—"there was no proof."

Today, 10 years after the [1989] fall of the Berlin Wall, it can be difficult to recall just how impregnable it once seemed. Like the Iron Curtain, it provided a blank canvas on which both East and West could project their failings and fears. Certainly that's what some critics thought athletes from rival nations were doing when they accused the East Germans of cheating. Unlike the Iron Curtain, however, the Berlin Wall didn't just stand for something. It stood. And when it fell, the piles of rubble provided not only a dramatic symbol for the collapse of Communism but something literal as well: a clear path toward information as concrete as the Wall itself.

Surviving evidence of doping

Despite the frantic efforts of party functionaries to shred decades' worth of evidence, hundreds of documents pertaining to the East German doping program survived. The Central Investigative Unit for Governmental Crimes and Crimes Relating to Reunification located a 10-volume file in the archives of Stasi, the East German secret police. More evidence came from the deputy director and chief physician of the national Sports Medical Service, Manfred Höppner, who sold key documents to the German magazine *Stern* in 1990.

The picture that emerged from these materials was specific, comprehensive, damning. One set of documents named more than 400 athletes and enumerated their secret chemical history—types of drugs, dosages, when they received them, even when they didn't receive them because they'd soon be competing internationally and subject to urine tests. Far more incriminating than the specific facts was the thorough accounting of the doping program itself.

The drugging of athletes began in the late '60s, in anticipation of the 1972 Olympics in Munich. The drug of choice was an anabolic steroid, Oral-Turanibol. Anabolic steroids are derivatives of testosterone that help during training rather than during competition by shortening the athlete's recovery time; they can improve a person's strength by more than 5 percent, especially among women, where a little testosterone goes proportionately farther than it does in men. As a result, wrote German biologist Werner Franke in the journal *Clinical Chemistry*, "Special emphasis was placed on administering androgens to women and adolescent girls."

Early results were more than promising. At the 1972 Olympics, East Germany, with its 20 gold medals, ranked third, behind the Soviet Union, with 50, and the United States, with 33. By the next year the authorities had developed a code name for the drug, Unterstützende Mittel, or "supporting means." "Under UM," wrote several prominent doctors and coaches in a secret report that introduced the euphemism, "we refer exclusively to anabolic steroids."

Since 1976, athletes from many countries have used the East German doping model.

On October 23, 1974, the Commission for High-Performance Sport, part of the Central Committee of the Socialist Party, approved State Plan Research Theme 14.25, the document that formalized the dissemination of performance-enhancing drugs to more than 2,000 athletes a year. By 1977, according to the deputy director of the Sports Medical Service, the reach of State Plan 14.25 was unambiguous: "At present anabolic steroids are applied in all Olympic sporting events, with the exception of sailing and gymnastics (female)." (The gymnastics restriction was lifted a year later.)

Even after the secret files on doping became public in the early '90s, some athletes didn't believe they had been drugged. Kornelia Ender said she couldn't be sure what was in the "vitamin cocktails" she'd downed every day. She went on to recall how her mother ("a nurse, after all") once had told her that maybe swimmers develop deep voices "because they are in the water all the time." Her father remembered confronting Kornelia's doctor at her swim club and telling him he didn't want his daughter taking drugs. "He told me that was none of my business," Ender's father told

Sports Illustrated in 1992. "He said that since I had agreed to Konni's performance goals, I should leave it up to them to prepare her properly." The father added that since he believed the doctor would have informed him if Konni had received drugs, it therefore hadn't happened.

In April 1974, the IOC voted to put anabolic steroids on the list of banned substances and to test for them at the 1976 Olympics. The East Germans now needed to figure out ways to counteract detection. Throughout the late '70s and early '80s, Manfred Höppner himself served on international drug commissions, which allowed him to monitor each new drug detection test and then pass the information on to East German sports authorities. As Werner Franke wrote, "in 1982, before the doping control test for testosterone administration was introduced, the doping scientists of the GDR had a solution." Even a positive result during an event posed no threat. Höppner routinely covered up positives and produced false negatives, and as the person responsible for transporting the tests, he could even "break the seals and exchange the urine samples," he wrote in one Stasi report.

Among themselves, swimmers began to refer to the East Germans as "bionic women."

For 20 years East Germany engaged in a systematic manipulation of human subjects through chemistry that was, as Franke once remarked, "reminiscent of the Third Reich." Still, the revelations didn't constitute legal proof. Then, in 1997, German prosecutors initiated two trials, accusing seven ex-coaches and two physicians of causing bodily harm to underage female swimmers between 1974 and 1989.

As prosecutors hoped, the publicity had a catalyzing effect on the athletes themselves. Two world swimming champions, Jörg Hoffman and Karen König, admitted that they had taken performance-enhancing drugs on a daily basis—little blue "vitamin" pills—during the '80s. "It was a ritual activity," said König, "like brushing your teeth." In what was to become a refrain at the two trials, Christiane Knacke-Sommer (then Knacke), a 1980 Olympic bronze medalist, testified that coaches had forcibly administered injections. Rica Reinisch, winner of three golds in 1980, blamed her ovarian cysts on hormones she'd unknowingly begun taking at age 12. Shotputter Heidi Krieger, the 1986 European champion, contended that her unwitting ingestion of male hormones had led to facial hair, an Adam's apple and her eventual decision to undergo a sex change. In 1997, Heidi announced that she was now Andreis and went into hiding.

The physical effects of the drugs were crucial to the government's case. Under German law, prosecutors had to prove not that the defendants had administered illegal drugs, nor that they had done so to minors (neither in itself is a crime in Germany), but that those drugs had caused bodily harm. According to Franke, the effects of male hormones on a woman athlete included severe acne, excessive genital hair, an enlarged clitoris, nymphomania and possible fetal damage if she became pregnant. In addition, the drugs could lead to kidney, liver and heart damage, as well as to femalelike breasts and enlarged nipples in men (there were 12 cases of breast amputation). One doctor testified that he had believed the effects of the hormones were reversible—if true, a tragic error.

Not all athletes cooperated with the investigations, and not all defendants confessed. Still, prosecutors managed to secure several key convictions (including one against Rolf Gläser, the "swim, not sing" coach), resulting in modest fines—and this, at last, was proof.

Response of American swimmers

How individual U.S. swimmers responded to the 1976 setbacks generally depended on what was at stake back then. Lauri Siering, now an assistant principal and mother, regards the events of her youth with some perspective. "It's taken me 20 years to get over the Olympics, twice as long as it took me to get there," she says. Camille Wright-Thompson, a mother of two, reflects, "The thing is, most of us did our best times, but sometimes your best isn't good enough." Ask Linda Wittwer if she often thinks back to 1976 and she replies, quickly, "No."

Yet among the women who were the wrong sex in the wrong sport at the wrong time, one name has always stood alone: Shirley Babashoff. Going into the 1976 Games, she had the most to lose, and she lost it. Her response to the East German winners at Montreal earned her a new nickname, "Surly Shirley," and a legacy as the anti-Spitz. Within a year, she retired, at age 20, and eventually she abandoned the water altogether. "If I fell into a pool," she once said, "I'd swim to the side." She married briefly in the late '70s, had a son by another man, worked odd jobs as a single mother and finally found steady employment as a mail carrier near her home, south of Los Angeles. Occasionally she would surface in some where-are-they-now? story ("Favorites Who Lost—How It Scarred Their Lives," read one headline) and dispense a one-liner about the 1976 Games: "What was I going to say—'Congratulations, you took the most steroids'?" But Babashoff's legacy is punch line enough: To this day her total of eight Olympic medals has been equaled by only two other swimmers—one of them, Kornelia Ender.

Then came the fall of the Berlin Wall, and with it the prospect of vindication. "I don't expect them to send me the medals," Babashoff said when the first files surfaced in the early '90s. "But I would like for them to say, 'We're going to change all the record books and make you the winner, because these people were on drugs.' That would make me feel good."

From the start of the trials, the USOC maintained that it would need a name before it could petition the IOC to amend the record books: one name to match one meet, the outcome of which might have been different if not for doping. Last year, the USOC got it: Andrea Pollack, one of the athletes prosecutors named in the case against the East German coaches and a member of the 400-meter medley relay team that had beaten Babashoff and company. The USOC arrived at the diplomatic solution of requesting not that the Germans give up their medals but that the Americans receive "appropriate medal recognition"—new medals or certificates, or even an asterisk in the record books. Last November the USOC sent letters notifying Shirley Babashoff, Lauri Siering, Linda Wittwer and Camille Wright-Thompson that it would present their case.

Siering, Wittwer and Wright-Thompson were excited. "I've got to be frank," said Siering. "I would be just tickled pink to get the gold."

And Babashoff? "Nothing is going to happen," she told a local reporter who caught up with her on her mail route. "To me, this happened a long time ago. It's like beating a dead horse. People have talked for 22 years." Of her Olympic medals, she added, "I'd sell them in a heartbeat for the right price."

For Babashoff, it's already too late. With the exception of that one interview, she has stopped talking to journalists (she didn't respond to several requests from *Women's Sports & Fitness*), stopped talking about swimming and, apparently, just stopped caring. In this regard at least, she and former archrival Kornelia Ender have finally found a common ground. When *Women's Sports & Fitness* reached Ender by telephone in Germany, she said, "I get upset at [this subject]. I don't want to talk about it. It's just unmöglich"—roughly translated, "tiresome."

Yet not every swimmer is content to consign that period of her life to fate. More than any of her teammates, Wendy Boglioli has fought for restitution. She swam the 100-meter butterfly and finished behind Ender and, yes, Pollack. Boglioli, a motivational speaker, doesn't swim any more but has taken up masters bicycle racing. Recently, she fell at a local velodrome, shattering her left arm in 16 places. Says Boglioli, "I look at Shirley: four silver medals? No. She should have had five gold medals. She was one of the best women athletes ever, and she deserves recognition."

Despite the evidence, several former East Germans quarrel with those who would rewrite history. "The biggest mistake we made," said former director Manfred Höppner, "was that we noted everything down conscientiously, and that is why we are now at the center of media attention, as though we had been the only ones who broke the rules of sport." Katarina Witt, the Olympic figure skating champion, told *The New York Times*, "Until everyone opens their files, I don't think it's fair to go after the Germans."

Doping in other countries

The truth is, since 1976, athletes from many countries have used the East German doping model: Twenty-seven Chinese swimmers have tested positive over the past decade, Irish swimmer Michelle Smith failed an out-of-competition drug test in 1998, and cyclists on the 1998 Dutch Tour de France cycling team tested positive for drugs. In addition to the high-profile cases of Canadian sprinter Ben Johnson and U.S. shot-putter Randy Barnes (banned for life for using drugs), 75 anonymous American athletes tested positive just before the 1984 Olympics (during a penalty-free testing period).

The USOC all but admits its own problem. Boglioli, who pestered the committee for years to take action on the 1976 case, says, "A top guy at the USOC, I won't mention his name, said to me, 'Wendy, you can't really keep pushing this, because we've got our own athletes on steroids. Now, how is it going to look if we point the finger? They're going to be looking at us, going, "Hey, you guys are doing it."' And I said, 'But isn't that the point?' I mean, why *are* our athletes doing it?"

And then she sighs, because she knows why: The punishment is too lax for a first-time offender: suspension rather than a lifetime ban.

("What is *that*?") The financial inducements are too tempting—$50,000 from USA Swimming for each gold medal, plus a onetime bonus of $15,000 from the USOC. ("*Hello*?") But the single most important factor in creating a system that rewards athletes who take drugs and officials who look the other way: sponsorships that are too lucrative.

If government-supported manipulation of body chemistry for the glory of the state was a hallmark of totalitarianism, then what is corporate-induced manipulation of body chemistry for the gain of the individual if not a hallmark of the free-market system? As Franke wrote, "only the extent and the pattern of organization differ essentially" between East and West. In the West, athletes might voluntarily dope themselves, but the competitive pressure is the same: sink or swim.

In the end, Shirley Babashoff was right. Nothing came of the USOC request. In December 1998 the IOC rejected the USOC petition, citing "too many variables involved to attempt to rewrite Olympic history." Bill Hybl, president of the USOC, says his organization will continue to pursue medal recognition through whatever means available. "We have not given up," he says. In the meantime, he's said he hopes the USOC can honor the cheated Americans with a "special banquet."

"Big deal!" says Boglioli. "It's an insult!" She laughs. "Yeah, I won't be going."

In February 1999 the IOC convened a World Conference on Doping in Sport. At the meeting, government and sports officials from around the world squabbled over penalties for athletes and openly castigated the leadership of the IOC. Yet, even in the face of such pressure, the IOC couldn't pass the two proposals it had convened the conference to consider: a mandatory two-year ban for testing positive and the creation of an independent antidoping agency. Meanwhile, the IOC insists it is pursuing refinements of drug testing and pledges to invest $25 million in an "antidoping police unit."

"Millions and millions of dollars testing athletes!" Boglioli says. "That could be money going into training facilities, school programs, and where does it go? To test the athletes because the athletes themselves don't have any integrity. I wish they would all get caught. Aren't we supposed to have honesty and passion and love of who we are and what we do, and grasp that and hold on to that? I mean, we stand up there and take an Olympic *oath*," and then she raises her broken left arm.

4

Performance-Enhancing Substances Raise Serious Ethical Questions for Athletes

Kirk Johnson

Kirk Johnson is a writer for the New York Times.

The substance androstenedione, a compound that can temporarily boost levels of the hormone testosterone, became famous when baseball player and home run slugger Mark McGwire admitted using it during the 1998 baseball season. McGwire's admission epitomizes how performance drugs in sports have become a matter of public knowledge and debate. Changes in federal law regulating food supplements have made androstenedione and similar substances readily and legally obtainable in the United States. But many people wonder whether using these substances is a way of cheating, and whether there should be more legal or ethical restrictions on using such substances.

Mark McGwire, the brawny St. Louis Cardinals first baseman, has become a folk hero to many people for his skill at hitting home runs, baseball's most dramatic—and clear-cut—feat. The ball flies out of the park, or it doesn't. But McGwire's recent admission [in August 1998] that he has used a testosterone-boosting compound for the . . . [previous] year has led him and his fans into a place where uncertainties abound.

The substance used by McGwire, called androstenedione and originally developed by East Germany's state-sponsored athletic drug program in the 1970's, in many ways epitomizes the new wave of performance drugs that is sweeping through the sports world, and its use underscores the ambiguities and questions that have arisen: What do these substances do? How can they be detected? Should they be legal? If they are legal, is it ethically right to take them? How should fans feel about athletes who do?

Last month [July 1998], the top team in the Tour de France was ex-

Reprinted from Kirk Johnson, "Performance Enhancing Drugs Proliferate, and So Do Ethical Questions," *The New York Times*, August 31, 1998. Reprinted with permission from *The New York Times*.

pelled after a team car was discovered to have a trunk-load of drugs, including a blood thickener and drugs that mask steroids. Earlier this month [August 1998], two former Olympic gold medalists from the United States, the shot-putter Randy Barnes and the sprinter Dennis Mitchell, were suspended by track and field's world governing body for suspected drug use. Members of the Chinese national swim team were banned earlier [in 1998] after vials of human growth hormone were seized in their possession. In all of those cases, the drugs were—unlike traditional anabolic steroids—not directly detectable by current lab tests.

Changes in federal law

The difficulty is compounded by big money and science, intertwined in the so-called natural supplement and additives industry that has arisen following Federal deregulation. The loosening of the laws dealing with food supplements—intended to encourage the market for herbal remedies and natural products—created an opening for products like androstenedione (pronounced an-dro-steen-DIE-own) which can be derived from things like the Mexican yam plant and the Scottish white pine. Manufacturers and medical experts say these products would not have been available over the counter under the old Food and Drug Administration rules.

By calling a substance a supplement and carefully avoiding any claims that it can cure a medical condition, a product can be labeled a food even though in most of the world it is a controlled substance.

"It's opened the door for a lot of people to push the limits of the law," Millard J. Baker said of the 1994 law. Baker is the founder and editor of *Mesomorphosis*, an on-line magazine that follows the supplement and muscle-building industry.

The changes in the law have also altered how the United States is regarded in the world sports community and have changed American attitudes, medical experts say, about products that might once have seemed risky, but which can now be purchased over the counter like vitamins or painkillers. Sports trainers and athletes say that what was once unthinkable has become common—foreign athletes are coming to the United States to buy performance-enhancing substances like androstenedione that are illegal in their home countries.

Meanwhile, other substances like creatine, an amino acid powder also said to help build muscles, have become as unremarkable as free weights in locker rooms from high school on up to professional teams. The Chicago Cubs' Sammy Sosa, who has been running neck and neck with McGwire in the race to break Roger Maris's single-season home run record, is one of many athletes who says he takes creatine. Creatine has not raised the same alarms as androstenedione, but physicians say its long-term effects are not known.

It all adds up to big profits. The supplement industry had $12 billion in sales last year [1997], up from $8 billion before the Federal law took effect, says *Nutrition Business Journal*, a trade publication.

The result is a multilevel conflict—for drug-detection labs and suppliers, each racing to keep ahead of the other; for athletes who are, as always, pressured to find and keep a competitive edge, and for fans who must decide what they want or do not want their sports heroes to be.

Conflicting claims and differing bans

Androstenedione is banned by the National Football League, the International Olympic Committee and the National Collegiate Athletic Association, which also ban all anabolic steroids. Federal law treats anabolic steroids as controlled substances, available only by prescription. Major League Baseball bans illegal drugs and a list of other substances, including anabolic steroids. The National Basketball Association currently has no drug policy that includes testing for steroids, and the National Hockey League bans only illegal drugs. General Nutrition Centers, one of the biggest retail chains, does not sell androstenedione because it says it is not yet convinced that it is safe.

"The line between what is effective and legal and what is effective and illegal is fading—it's not clear anymore because the people who are making these other substances are getting very good and they are finding ways to dim the line," said Harold Connolly, a former Olympic hammer-thrower and world record-holder who used steroids in the 1960's before coming out against their use.

The man generally regarded as the father of androstenedione production in United States—an Illinois chemist named Patrick Arnold, who translated German medical documents and patents in the mid-1990's after the fall of the Soviet Union—said he thinks the product is safe when taken correctly. Unlike traditional steroids, which can make testosterone levels soar to dangerous levels, so-called precursor substances like androstenedione are converted to testosterone within the body. Arnold said he thinks the body can create only so much testosterone by this method and no more—the rest, he said, simply gets washed out.

What was once unthinkable has become common— foreign athletes are coming to the United States to buy . . . substances . . . that are illegal in their home countries.

"If you take more, you cannot breach this ceiling, so far as we can tell," said Arnold, who created the first commercial batches in the United States in 1996. "You will not reach superphysiological levels."

Now the news about McGwire and the confusion about whether scientists like Arnold are correct seem to have sparked efforts to reconsider the new compounds and the supplement industry in general.

Major League Baseball and its players' union said they would look at the medical and performance aspects. The International Olympic Committee proposed setting up an agency to coordinate drug testing around the world. The Association of Professional Team Physicians, made up of doctors from most major league sports in the United States, this week [in August 1998] called on baseball to denounce and ban androstenedione. [Editor's note: As of September 2000 Major League Baseball has not officially banned androstenedione. McGwire announced in 1999 that he was no longer using it.]

Meanwhile, sales of health and performance-enhancement products have surged from the publicity, and companies are racing ahead with new products. Met-Rx, a company in Irvine, California, with which Arnold is affiliated, said that it was developing a gum that boosted testosterone—three times more effectively than the stuff McGwire takes, company officials boasted—while you chew. Another company has developed a steroid that dissolves under the tongue. Advertising copy on the Internet bursts with claims about everything from better state of mind to heightened sexual performance.

Ethical questions

But there is much more than pharmacology to the McGwire story. In many ways, McGwire's testing of his own limits at the plate has become a test for Americans in general, experts in ethics and sports say.

Should there be limits, either in morality or law, on how much and through what means an individual can improve upon fate or genes? Should enhancement efforts for athletes be considered differently from the efforts of ordinary people to improve their states of mind through drugs like Prozac, their sexual performance with drugs like Viagra or their hairlines with drugs like Propecia? What, in a time of exploding interest and economic growth in natural herbal substances and medicines, is a drug? What does the term "natural" even mean?

Many drug monitors say that as testing has improved, "natural" substances—harder to detect in the body, and with a legal base of operations under the Federal food supplement law—have become the last refuge for cheaters.

"In today's world, athletes who are determined to cheat know that natural substances are the way to go," said Dr. Don H. Catlin, a professor of medicine and pharmacology at U.C.L.A. and a member of the medical commission of the I.O.C., which specifically banned androstenedione late last year [1997]. Catlin said many newer substances, including androstenedione, cannot be detected by current tests and are new enough that many leagues have not formed policies about their use—which makes them attractive to athletes on multiple levels. "And there's a whole cornucopia of other things right behind it," Catlin said. "That's where things are going."

Compounding the questions is that McGwire, in chasing one of the most hallowed records in sports, has tapped into a vein of romance and nostalgia for a supposedly sunnier, more innocent time.

"I think this taps some pretty deep roots about what sport means to us—because it's baseball and baseball has a special place in the American psyche," said Tom Murray, the director of the Center for Biomedical Ethics at Case Western Reserve University and a member of the anti-doping committee of the United States Olympic Committee. "Ultimately, this is a question about values. I think people are really struggling with it."

Confusing message to young athletes

Most awkwardly, perhaps, people are struggling with what to tell young people, both about what is safe and about what, if anything, it means that a star like McGwire, a man with a wealth of positive attributes, looks for a controversial edge.

"Instead of telling kids not to take it, he comes out and says, in effect, 'It's O.K. because it's allowed,'" said Dr. Lewis G. Maharam, the president of the New York chapter of the American College of Sports Medicine. "He needs to say, 'What I'm doing for me is my business, but for you kids, there's evidence that this stuff is like steroids—listen to your doctors and don't be buying it.'"

Some professional athletes, while not criticizing McGwire for his supplement use, say he has to be careful because so many kids hang on his every word and deed.

"There's a lot of kids out there who think that if the home run king is doing it, then I should be doing it," said Mark Jackson, the Indiana Pacers point guard. "It's time for him to put out his own warning label for the kids of America, to tell them that no one knows the long-term effects of what he is using and it could prove to be harmful."

Many baseball fans, including parents of young children, say that they are willing to give McGwire the benefit of the doubt.

"I don't fault him for trying to enhance his performance," said Larry Rhine, a chiropractor from Allentown, Pennsylvania, who was in Williamsport, Pennsylvania, with his 8-year-old son, Mark, watching the Little League World Series. "If he's within the legal bounds of Major League Baseball, it shouldn't taint him at all." Rhine said his son did not seem to be having any second thoughts either: Mark still got up every morning eager to see if McGwire or Sosa had hit another home run, Rhine said.

Arnold, the chemist, agreed in an interview that no one under 18 should think of using androstenedione. He said that the company he works with, Met-Rx, is careful to put such warnings on its products. But he admitted that the implications of such use are largely unknown. A 16-year-old male, for example, whose body is already producing a bumper crop of testosterone, probably would not be harmed by taking the compound, Arnold said.

"But it's sort of an unknown," he added.

Companies that sell supplements say that business has never been better. Chico Laney, who started a mail-order supplement company, Muscle Up, out of his parents' house in San Jose, California, three months ago [in May 1998], said that before the McGwire story broke, sales were slow—sometimes only one order a week. Over the past week, however, he had received six to seven orders a day, mainly for androstenedione, which he gets from an Oregon manufacturer.

Laney said that at least one of the calls was from a 45-year-old man who had heard that boosting testosterone would cure impotence. Laney said he was not sure, because he really did not know himself what androstenedione would do.

"I didn't guarantee that it was going to do that," Laney said. "I told him to call back, because I'd be curious to know."

5

The International Olympic Committee Stands Against Doping

Juan Antonio Samaranch

Juan Antonio Samaranch is president of the International Olympic Committee, a private organization that supervises the organizing of the Olympic Games.

Doping is a danger for the health of athletes and a mockery of the ideals of sport and of the Olympic Movement. The International Olympic Committee has sought to ban the use of drugs in sports and to collaborate with national sports federations, organizations, and governments in this endeavor.

The International Olympic Committee has always endeavoured to adapt, as best it can, to the constantly changing conditions of the fight against doping. Alas, the tinkerers of sports performance are forever searching to find new methods, often assisted by specialists who attach little importance to the code of ethics they are supposed to respect.

Doping is not only a danger for the health of athletes, it also constitutes a form of cheating which we cannot accept. Apparently, the desire to win at all costs drives some to turn to illegal and totally unfair means in order to ensure that the athletes in their charge gain an advantage over their rivals. As means of detection have improved, they now attempt to cheat scientifically by artificially inducing natural physiological reactions, or by attempting with various tricks to hide the evidence of these manipulations.

It will come as no surprise to anyone that, as IOC President and custodian of the entire Olympic Movement, I am taking such a serious and firm stand against these practices. Such an attitude, and such behaviour, constitute in and of themselves very serious violations of the sporting laws, prescribed in the first instance by the IOC and by a growing number of International sports Federations, National Olympic Committees,

Reprinted from Juan Antonio Samaranch, "The Fight Against Doping," an undated article found at www.nodoping.org/pos_samar_e.html. Reprinted with permission from the author and the International Olympic Committee.

and indeed by governments themselves. But above all, such behaviour makes a mockery of the very essence of sport, and of the soul of what our predecessors, like ourselves, consider to be sacrosanct ideals: the inner desire to surpass one's own limits, the social need to compete with others, to find one's identity within society and to develop at all levels.

> *Doping is not only a danger for the health of athletes, it also constitutes a form of cheating which we cannot accept.*

Many hundreds of millions of players freely accept our principles and share our ideals, and we absolutely reject these attempts to cheat, which endanger the health and the very lives of those involved. We were the first, starting in 1968, to assume responsibility for the fight against the use of doping substances, and we intend fully to carry on, in close collaboration with the International sports Federations, the National Olympic Committees, and inter- and non-governmental organizations.

We know that this will be a long and constantly changing battle, necessitating close cooperation among all who bear responsibility for the education and well-being of youth. For this reason, the IOC is organizing, from 2 to 4 February 1999, a World Conference on Doping in Sport, so that all the parties concerned can reflect and make a firmer commitment to the fight against doping, which is poisoning the world of sport. We have already won several battles, but we have not yet won the war.

6

The Impropriety of Taking Performance-Enhancing Drugs Is Debatable

Gina Kolata

Gina Kolata is a science reporter for the New York Times.

Scandals involving performance-enhancing drugs are a recurring issue in the athletic world. However, some medical ethicists have questioned why drug use is so readily condemned by those who applaud other "unnatural" methods of improving one's athletic performance, such as altitude training and special diets. They argue that the use of drugs as a training and performance aid should be an individual decision left up to the athletes.

It happened again this year [1999]. Another drug scandal in sports. This time, it involved more than a dozen cyclists in Swiss and Italian races failing blood tests, including Marco Pantani of Italy, last year's winner of the Tour de France.

But some critics are pointing to what they see as a disconnect between excessive worry over performance-enhancing drugs and uncritical applause for the other ways of boosting an athlete's performance—from high-technology running shoes to chains of stores devoted to dietary supplements.

The laments over the cycling scandal sounded all too familiar to anyone who has followed the continuing drama of drugs in sports. A common reaction is often disgust. Daniel Baal, the president of the French Cycling Federation, said with drug use so rampant, "I can't watch a fake spectacle."

If an athlete excels—or develops an injury or illness—charges of drug use spring up. European cycling officials charged the athletes with using erythropoietin, or EPO, which raises red blood cell counts, enabling the blood to carry more oxygen to muscles. Now, when cyclists sprint up a mountain flawlessly, spectators may well ask: Is it natural ability combined with tough training? Or is it EPO?

In the July 1996 issue of the *Journal of the American Medical Associa-*

Reprinted from Gina Kolata, "Slippery Slope on the Playing Field," *The New York Times*, July 11, 1999. Reprinted with permission from *The New York Times*.

tion, Dr. Thomas Murray, the president of the Hastings Center, an ethics institute, and Dr. Don Catlin, who operates the Olympic drug-testing lab at the University of California at Los Angeles, wrote that drug testing in the Olympics "is an effort to preserve what is beautiful and admirable in sports and to ensure that all athletes compete on a level playing field."

But some critics argue that drug use is not inherently different from other ways many top athletes try to gain that tiny margin that separates the winners from the losers.

A double standard?

Take the arguments surrounding EPO. Dr. Norman Fost, the director of the program in medical ethics at the University of Wisconsin and an outspoken critic of what he sees as a double standard, says there are three ways to raise the hemoglobin level of blood: Train at high altitudes or spend time in chambers with low oxygen levels, which accomplishes the same thing. Bank your own red blood cells and then inject them. Or take EPO.

"What's hypocritical is saying there's something immoral about using mechanism three or mechanism two," Dr. Fost said.

Yet many argue that taking a drug like EPO is unnatural. What does it mean to break a world record when the athlete's edge is supplied by a drug as opposed to something else? "Tell me a sport or show me an athlete that doesn't have unnatural assists," Dr. Fost said, referring not only to special running shoes and fiberglass poles for pole vaults but also to secret devices and methods.

Drugs are chemicals that change the body, but so are special training diets.

When the American swimmer Janet Evans won a gold medal in the 1988 Olympics in Seoul, she wore a "slime suit," a greasy swimsuit that had been developed in secret, which slashed her time. At that same Olympics, the Canadian sprinter Ben Johnson was stripped of his gold medal because he had failed a test for steroids. Dr. Fost says Ms. Evans won praise for using an unnatural assist while Mr. Johnson was vilified.

Drugs are chemicals that change the body, but so are special training diets, says Michael Shapiro, a law professor at the University of Southern California. So is Gatorade. "One of the feelings about drugs is that they somehow make the athlete superhuman, as opposed to getting a better bicycle or a better pole vault," said James Bakalar, the associate editor of the *Harvard Mental Health Letter.* "When you analyze this, it doesn't work out too clearly."

Drugs and risk

But aren't such performance-enhancing drugs dangerous? They are certainly perceived to be. If spectacular victories raise suspicions about drugs, so do illnesses. When the American sprinter Florence Griffith Joyner, the winner of three gold medals in the 1988 Olympics, died suddenly last year [1998] at age 38 of suffocation related to an epileptic seizure, there was a spate of unfounded whispers that drugs had killed her.

In a similar example, Dr. Murray writes in a 1983 article for The Hastings Center Report: "I have heard reports of two women, world champions in the 1970's, who appeared to age with stunning rapidity. While no conclusive proof is possible that these effects were due to steroids, or even that these two women used steroids, their women competitors have no doubt that steroids were the cause."

But the evidence that athletes were harmed by such drugs is scanty at best, said Dr. Fost. And if people are worried about physical impairment, he adds, the risks of taking drugs pale in comparison to the risks of simply playing many of the sports, even non-contact sports.

"Greg Louganis cracked his head on the diving platform," [in the 1988 Olympics] Dr. Fost said. "We didn't say we want to ban diving because of its danger."

What about the coercive nature of drugs, the pressure athletes may feel to use them to keep up with their competitors? By using drugs, athletes "have turned a sport into a sophisticated game of chicken," Dr. Murray writes.

No one has to take such drugs and most athletes refuse them, critics say. Yet every athlete takes part in a game of chicken when it comes to deprivation and risk in training.

Dr. Fost says there is perhaps another reason why drugs remain such a major issue in sports: They can be a welcome diversion from other issues, like the serious risks of permanent injury in football, gymnastics and other events. The drug issue, he said, is "a cheap fix, a way of appearing concerned about ethical problems in sports."

7

Drug Testing for Athletes Must Be Improved

Domhnall MacAuley

Domhnall MacAuley is editor of the British Journal of Sports Medicine *and the author of* Sports Medicine: Practical Guidelines for General Practice.

Many athletes, under great pressure to win by any means, seek a competitive advantage through drugs. The taking of drugs endangers the health of athletes and the principles of fair competition. Detecting such drug use has become increasingly difficult as new drugs and methods of cheating on drug tests have been developed. Countries and sports organizations should redouble their efforts to standardize drug testing procedures and make them more effective.

The use of drugs to enhance performance in sport will not go away. Athletes seek every competitive advantage and the rewards of success at top level are great, both financially and in personal glory. Almost all top level competitors are full time and, even if not paid, are to all purposes professional. There is huge pressure to train longer and harder and to take a scientific approach to nutrition and fluid and electrolyte balance, to seek every biomechanical and psychological advantage. It is almost inevitable that some will seek an advantage through drugs. Though there may be little clear objective scientific evidence of a benefit to be gained from drug use, what evidence there is supports the widespread belief among athletes that drugs help. Indeed, many believe that it is impossible to succeed without drugs. Though an athlete's motivation in taking drugs is understandable, we cannot condone it. Firstly, it can be dangerous to the athlete's health and, secondly, it is against all principles of fair competition.

An underground activity

A systematic search of the literature is unlikely to tell the complete story in any review of drug abuse in sport. Doping in sport is essentially an un-

Reprinted from Domhnall MacAuley, "Drugs in Sports," *British Medical Journal*, July 27, 1996. Reprinted with permission from BMJ Publishing Group.

derground activity with little formal published research in a topic which should not officially exist. Much of what is common knowledge is cloaked in rumour, suspicion, and suggestion, and the strategies adopted by athletes seem to be founded more on empiricism than published scientific data.

The information presented in this review has been identified from several sources. A Medline search from 1966 to 1996 identified 620 references to the term "doping in sports." With the search restricted to humans (504) and to publications in English there were 389 references. Those references were subclassified into publications identifying side effects, prevalence, methods of detection, and a fourth group composed of editorials, opinions, and reviews. Further references were identified from a search of the National Sports Medicine Institute database and a hand search of the past five years of the *British Journal of Sports Medicine.* Additional information is available from the annual report of the Sports Council [of the United Kingdom][1] and advisory booklets from the same source.[2, 3, 4, 5, 6, 7]

Classes of banned substances

Drugs prohibited by the International Olympic Committee include those listed below.

Stimulants. Amphetamines are used by athletes to increase aggression and competitiveness and to reduce tiredness and fatigue and have a long history of abuse, particularly in cycling. Adverse medical side effects may include a rise in blood pressure and body temperature, arrhythmias, aggression, anxiety, and addiction. Caffeine[8] is slightly unusual owing to its widespread social use and presence in many beverages. There is a threshold level and the concentration of caffeine in the urine should not exceed 12 µg/ml [micrograms/milliliter]. One group that causes particular problems is the sympathomimetic amines, of which ephedrine, pseudoephedrine, phenyl-propranolamine, and norpseudoephedrine are examples. These remain on the prohibited list, though doubts remain about their ergogenic [performance-related] effect.

Narcotic analgesics. Narcotic analgesics reduce pain sensitivity and enable an athlete to continue despite injury. Adverse effects of cocaine abuse have been recorded in athletes. Recent changes in the International Olympic Committee doping regulations mean that codeine, dihydrocodeine, and pholcodine are now permitted analgesics; it should be noted, however, that dextropropoxyphene remains a prohibited substance.

Anabolic steroids. Anabolic steroids are probably the best known drugs of abuse, though the evidence for their effectiveness had not been convincing[9] until the recent publication of a randomised controlled trial with high dose testosterone.[10] Side effects are well documented. They include psychological and psychiatric conditions, rupture of the musculocutaneous junction, gynaecomastia, hypogonadism, effects on coagulation and lipids and lipoproteins, cholestasis, skin disease, hypertension, stroke, and myocardial infarction. Chemical structures have been modified to increase the anabolic effect and reduce the androgenic effect and more than 100 different anabolic steroids are available, taken either by mouth or by injection. Most often used for their anabolic or muscle building effect, they also affect mood and aggression, which enables people to train harder.

Classically anabolic steroids are taken by power athletes, so are widely used and abused by body builders and recreational weight trainers, but they are also reputedly used as a training aid by endurance athletes to improve recovery from training loads. Doses greatly exceed the normal therapeutic doses and athletes may take several different types of anabolic steroid together (stacking) or vary the use of different steroids (cycling). Because these drugs are used essentially as training aids athletes may stop some weeks before an event and later pass the competition dope test. Clearly, if athletes knew their own clearance time for a particular oral or injectable drug they could plan drug use to give the maximum benefit with least risk of detection. Other drugs used concurrently may include diuretics to reduce fluid retention, thyroxine to promote weight loss, and tamoxifen to prevent gynaecomastia. These agents are quite freely available in gymnasiums and fitness clubs throughout Britain.

Because of the difficulties in testing for testosterone the testosterone to epitestosterone ratio is used as the clue to detection. ß2 [Beta$_2$] agonists used systemically also have powerful anabolic effects, hence clenbuterol is banned. Other ß2 agonists are also prohibited, though salbutamol, salmeterol, and terbutaline, which are prohibited for systemic use, are permitted by inhalation if previously declared. Doubts remain about the possibility of false positive test results,[11] and indeed a recent paper examined the effect on drug tests of eating meat from steroid treated livestock.[12]

ß [Beta] blockers. ß [Beta] blockers are used both to control the effects of anxiety and, in some sports—notably shooting[13] and archery—to produce bradycardia. In these sports and others in which accuracy and control are important, such as bowls, ß blockers have great potential effect; but they are clearly of little use in physically active sports. Other sports in which the use of ß blockers is banned include bobsleigh and luge, ski jumping and free style skiing, diving and synchronised swimming, and modern pentathlon.

Diuretics. Diuretics have been abused in those sports in which athletes compete at weight limits and are used to shed weight quickly. They have also been used to increase urine volume and dilution to make detection of small quantities of banned substances more difficult.

Peptide hormones. Peptide hormones, the so called sports designer drugs, may be used for several reasons. Their main attraction from the athlete's viewpoint is the difficulty of detection. Human growth hormone is used for its anabolic effect. The possibility that some growth hormone preparations of human origin may be associated with Creutzfeldt-Jacob disease has caused anxiety among some athletes. Corticotrophin increases the level of endogenous corticosteroids and may alter mood. Human chorionic gonadotrophin is used to increase the production of endogenous steroids.

"Blood doping." Athletes have always been aware of the possible benefit of improving oxygen carrying capacity in endurance sport, hence many train at altitude. More recently athletes have used blood doping—in which blood is taken off, stored, and later reinfused, thereby boosting the packed cell volume. Blood doping, which is effective,[14] is banned but exceptionally difficult to detect. It does, however, carry all the logistical

problems associated with storage and reinfusion in less than ideal conditions. Erythropoietin, initially developed to counter severe anaemia in renal failure, has been used by athletes as a more convenient method of increasing the packed cell volume. Its use is banned but currently undetectable. It is suspected but unproved that the sudden and unexplained death of some endurance athletes may be associated with the uncontrolled use of erythropoietin.

Manipulation of procedures and other drugs. Pharmacological, chemical, and physical manipulation of the drug testing procedure is also prohibited. This includes physical methods such as catheterisation, urine substitution, and tampering with samples. It also includes methods to inhibit renal excretion—for example, by using probenecid and related substances. Using epitestosterone to correct the ratio to testosterone is also prohibited.

Certain other drugs are subject to restriction. They include alcohol, marijuana, and local anaesthetics. Certain local anaesthetics are permitted for local or intra-articular use, and then only when medically justified and with prior notification to the relevant medical authority. Corticosteroids are permitted for topical use only (by inhalation and intra-articular and local injection), and then only with written notification to the relevant medical authority.

The problems

We can immediately identify the two main problems of drug control in sport. Some athletes deliberately take performance enhancing drugs and set out to avoid being caught. Others may inadvertently take a substance, even some without performance enhancing effect, and face censure because of a positive drug test result. These factors have major implications for athletes, doctors, and the organisation of the drug testing procedure.

Drug testing, or dope testing, is performed in almost all sports, and sports bodies faced with policing drug abuse publish lists of banned substances. These are substances believed to give the athlete some advantage, though not all prohibited drugs have a proved ergogenic effect. The list is huge and cannot be comprehensive, as many only slightly dissimilar drugs can have similar effect. The only way athletes can remain completely certain that they have not taken a prohibited substance is either to avoid all drugs or to take only those agents on the permitted list. This is not always easy.

Drugs available both on prescription and "over the counter" to treat common conditions such as catarrh or nasal congestion, and even some apparently innocuous preparations for pain relief, may contain banned substances. In addition, athletes who take health food supplements or vitamin products may inadvertently take prohibited substances, especially if these are purchased abroad, as labelling and lists of contents may be imprecise. For example, contents may not be listed on the package, the athlete may not recognise a banned substance, or the name may be colloquial, which may be misleading. Commonly available "over the counter" preparations that do contain a prohibited substance include products such as Bronchipax, Contac 400, Mucron, Nirolex expectorant, and Procol. These are only examples and many other drugs contain substances prohibited in sport.

Information sources for doctors and athletes

The Sports Council offers an information system so that athletes may find out about various agents and help protect themselves against the inadvertent use of a banned substance. Several booklets are available direct from the Sports Council. In addition, there is a hotline number (0171 383 2244) that athletes can use if they require a rapid response. At present this number is linked to an answering machine and the call is returned later. Plans are in hand to offer a direct access line. [Editor's note: information on contacting the Sports Council can be found in the organization list at the end of this book.] Even then it will be difficult to supply completely up to date and accurate information. Different sports may have different regulations and while some substances may be banned by one organisation they may be permitted by another. Athletes may be given advice but ultimately may be referred back to their own organisation, as providing a comprehensive list of banned substances for every sport is difficult.

How great is the problem?

We do not know the magnitude of the problem. We do know, however, the number of positive test results detected by the Sports Council's London testing laboratory (table 1) and note the rising numbers. Data are also available from the games of the 23rd Olympiad in Los Angeles,[15] where 1.7% of 1510 samples contained a banned drug. In 1986 at the 10th Asian games 3.2% of samples were found to contain a banned drug,[16] and at the 1988 winter Olympics 2.6% of test results were positive.[17] We also have data from dope testing in South Africa,[18] where during 1986–91, 5.5% of 2066 urine specimens collected from competitors contained drugs classified as forbidden by the International Olympic Committee.

Table 1: Results of dope testing (drug control centre, King's College, London)

Year	No. of tests	No. of positive tests	No. of refusals
1992	4167	48	10
1993	3946	41	6
1994	4374	67	7
1995	4596	84	15

Data from annual report of Sports Council, 1995–6.[1]

The problem seems to be greatest among body builders. In West Glamorgan Perry et al looked at anabolic steroid use in private gymnasiums and found that 38.8% of respondents admitted to having taken steroids.[19] In the west of Scotland 19.5% of body builders had used drugs to enhance their physique and performance.[20] In unannounced doping control among body builders in Flanders during 1988–93 between 38% and 58% of those tested were found to be positive during this period,[21] and in a study from the United States over half of the male body builders (54%) were using steroids regularly as compared with 10% of the female competitors.[22]

Though an athlete's motivation in taking drugs is understandable, we cannot condone it.

Even more worrying are figures from the United States, where the prevalence of steroid use among adolescents in large surveys has been found to be between 3.0% and 7.6%.[23, 24, 25, 26] Even human growth hormone abuse seems to be a problem in high schools, where 5% (n=11) of boys reported past or present use and 31% reported knowing someone who was using growth hormone.[27]

What do athletes think?

In February 1995 the Sports Council surveyed senior competitors from 26 winter and summer sports.[28] There was a 60% response rate (468). Though 74% had been tested at some point in their career and 66% thought it likely that they would be tested in the next 12 months, 34% expressed dissatisfaction at the range of competitors selected for testing and 41% expressed dissatisfaction about the frequency of testing. Many thought that testing should be more widespread and more often. About 70% believed that testing served as a deterrent, but a quarter believed that lack of widespread testing made the process less of a deterrent for some.

In a study of 1015 Italian athletes over 10% indicated a frequent use of amphetamines or anabolic steroids at national or international level, fewer athletes mentioning blood doping (7%) and ß blockers (2%) or other classes of drugs.[29] According to over 70% of athletes, access to illegal substances was not difficult. Eighty-two per cent wanted stricter controls not only during competitions but also during training.

Drug testing procedure

The drug testing procedure is as easy as taking a urine sample. This sounds deceptively simple, as testing is a formal and highly regulated procedure to ensure that the urine sample which arrives at the laboratory actually comes from the athlete in question, with no opportunity to tamper with the sample. When selected for testing the athlete is notified by an official and asked to sign a form acknowledging this notification. The athlete, who may be accompanied by an official and must be accompanied if under 16, attends the testing station within a stipulated period. The testing station should be a private, comfortable place where plenty of drinks are available; often it may be situated in a specially designed mobile testing caravan. Testing is carried out by independent sampling officers, trained and appointed by the Sports Council. Each carries a time limited identity card and a letter of authority for the event to which he or she is allocated.

Before giving a sample the athlete is invited to choose a set of two numbered bottles. Having given the sample (about 100 ml) the athlete completes a form on a voluntary basis declaring any drug treatment taken in the previous seven days and must check and sign that the sample has been taken and placed in the bottles correctly. The sample is then sent for analysis to a laboratory currently accredited by the International Olympic Committee. In the event of a positive test result the laboratory will notify the governing body of the sport, who will then notify the athlete. What happens then depends on the rules of the governing body of the particular sport. An athlete is usually suspended while a positive result is investigated but has the right to have a second analysis of the urine sample. This analysis may be observed by the athlete himself or herself or by the athlete's representative. There follows a hearing, at which the athlete has an opportunity to present his or her case. It is also possible to appeal, and there have been successful appeals both in the United Kingdom and in the United States.

The testing procedure is of necessity rigorous. Because drugs are potentially such a boost to performance athletes who use them they will go to great lengths not to be caught. Thus not only are various agents banned but other manipulative procedures are also banned. These include both mechanical and chemical methods. To ensure that the sample actually comes from the athlete the testing officer must be able to see the urine issue from the meatus and pass into the bottle. This is not quite as easy as it sounds. Male athletes must be stripped to the waist with their shorts to their knees. Female athletes must also be observed very closely during testing. There are many legends of athletes using elaborate arrangements of catheters to provide an alternative sample, bringing condoms filled with drug free urine to the testing station, and even catheterising themselves and instilling drug free urine. If athletes will go to these lengths to avoid detection the testing procedure must be strict and must be enforced.

Drug testing, or dope testing, is performed in almost all sports.

Clearly, however, this procedure may cause embarrassment. It can be upsetting for young athletes, perhaps in their late teens, just breaking through into the top national or international level, to give a urine sample under these circumstances. Indeed, many people are very uncomfortable being observed giving a urine sample. If, in addition, an athlete has been competing in an endurance sport and is dehydrated or competing at a weight category where he or she is reluctant to drink excess fluid we can appreciate how daunting it can be. It is equally important that athletes should ensure that the testing procedure is observed rigorously for their own protection, that their samples are dispatched in the correct containers, and that all the paperwork is completed with no chance of error. Once a sample is taken there must be a completely secure passage until it arrives in the laboratory.

Elite athletes are subject to year round random testing. Thus an independent sampling officer may call unannounced at any time and request a drug sample. Apparently quite straightforward, there may be organisational difficulties. Many of the most successful athletes travel the world freely and spend periods at warm weather training camps or at altitude. Sometimes finding the athlete can be difficult, and with all the necessary preliminary inquiries it is unlikely that the testing will remain a surprise.

The unpleasant necessity of drug testing

The only entirely safe way for an athlete to avoid prohibited substances is not to take drugs. There is, however, an overwhelming belief that drugs enhance performance and an athlete may believe that some drug must be taken to level the playing field; hence performance enhancing drugs have been described as coercive drugs.[30]

Can drug taking be stopped? The inevitable answer is that it cannot and that some athletes will always try to seek some extra competitive advantage. Drug taking can be controlled only if detection is likely and the penalties of detection are a sufficient deterrent. Unless there is widespread testing, both in and out of competition, the risk to benefit ratio favours the drug taker. There are therefore considerable difficulties in preventing the use of performance enhancing drugs. There should also, however, be protection for the athlete who inadvertently takes a prohibited substance, and because of the huge implications of a positive test result great care must be taken to avoid having false positive results.

Unless there is widespread testing, both in and out of competition, the risk to benefit ratio favours the drug taker.

Drug testing is unpleasant but seems to be here to stay. There will always be rumours of undetectable drugs, masking agents, or surgical procedures to subvert the dope test. And always there is the fear that the testers are one step behind and will never quite catch up.

I thank Michele Verroken, of the Sports Council Doping Control Unit; Stephen Martin, of the Sports Council for Northern Ireland; Yasmin Hossain, at the National Sports Medicine Institute of the United Kingdom; and the librarians at the British Medical Association for their help in the preparation of this paper.

Notes

1. Sports Council Doping Control Service. Report 1995–96. London: Sports Council, 1996.

2. Sports Council Doping Control Unit. Anabolic steroids. London: Sports Council, 1993. (Information booklet No 1.)

3. Sports Council Doping Control Unit. International Olympic Committee doping classes. London: Sports Council, 1994. (Information booklet No 2.)

4. Sports Council Doping Control Unit. International Olympic Committee accredited laboratories. London: Sports Council, 1994. (Information booklet No 3.)

5. Sports Council Doping Control Unit. Guide to allowable medications. London: Sports Council, 1995. (Information booklet No 4.)

6. Sports Council Doping Control Unit. Suggested further reading. London: Sports Council, 1994. (Information booklet No 5.)

7. Sports Council Doping Control Unit. UK legislation on doping substances. London: Sports Council, 1993. (Information booklet No 6.)

8. Spriet LL. Caffeine and performance. International Journal of Sport Nutrition 1995;5(suppl):S84–99.

9. Elashoff JD, Jacknow AD, Shain SG, Braunstein GD. Effects of anabolic-androgenic steroids on muscular strength. *Ann Intern Med* 1991;115:387–93.

10. Bhasin S, Storer TW, Berman N, Callegari C, Clevenger B, Phillips J, et al. The effects of supraphysiologic doses of testosterone on muscle size and strength in normal men. *N Engl J Med* 1996;335:1–7.

11. Raynaud E, Audran M, Brun JF, Fedou C, Chanal JL, Orsetti A. False-positive cases in detection of testosterone doping. *Lancet* 1992;340:1468–9.

12. Kicman AT, Cowan DA, Myhre L, Nilsson S, Tomten S, Oftebro H. Effect on sports drug tests of ingesting meat from steroid- (methenolone)- treated livestock. *Clin Chem* 1994;40:2084–7.

13. Kruse P, Ladefoged J, Nielsen, Paulev PE, Sorensen JP. Beta-blockade used in precision sports: effects on pistol shooting performance. *J Appl Physiol* 1986;61:417–20.

14. Berglund B, Hemmingson P. Effect of reinfusion of autologous blood on exercise performance in cross-country skiers. *Int J Sports Med* 1987;8:231–3.

15. Catlin DH, Kammerer RC, Hatton CK, Sekera MH, Merdink JL. Analytical chemistry at the games of the XXIIIrd Olympiad in Los Angeles, 1984. *Clin Chem* 1987;33:319–27.

16. Park J. Doping test report of 10th Asian games in Seoul. *J Sports Med Phys Fitness* 1991;31:303–17.

17. Chan SC, Torok-Both GA, Billay DM, Przybylski PS, Gradeen CY, Pap KM, et al. Drug analysis at the 1988 Olympic Winter Games in Calgary. *Clin Chem* 1991;37:1289–96.

18. van der Merwe PJ, Kruger HS. Drugs in sport—results of the past 6 years of dope testing. *South Afr Med J* 1992;82:151–3.

19. Perry HM, Wright D, Littlepage BN. Dying to be big: a review of anabolic steroid use. *Br J Sports Med* 1992;26:259–61.

20. McKillop G. Drug abuse in body builders in the west of Scotland. *Scott Med J* 1987;32:39–41.

21. Delbeke FT, Desmet N, Debackere M. The abuse of doping agents in competing body builders in Flanders (1988–1993). *Int J Sports Med* 1995;16: 66–70.

22. Tricker R, O'Neill MR, Cook D. The incidence of anabolic steroid use among competitive bodybuilders. *J Drug Educ* 1989;19:313–25.

23. Whitehead R, Chillag S, Elliott D. Anabolic steroid use among adolescents in a rural state. *J Fam Pract* 1992;35:401–5.

24. Komoroski EM, Rickert VI. Adolescent body image and attitudes to anabolic steroid use. *Am J Dis Child* 1992;146:823–8.

25. Terney R, McLain LG. The use of anabolic steroids in high school students. *Am J Dis Child* 1990;144:99–103.

26. Windsor R, Dumitru D. Prevalence of anabolic steroid use by male and female adolescents. *Med Sci Sports Exerc* 1989;21:494–7.

27. Rickert VI, Pawlak-Morello C, Sheppard V, Jay MS. Human growth hormone: a new substance of abuse among adolescents? *Clin Pediatr* 1992;31:723–6.

28. Sports Council. Doping control in the UK. A survey of the experiences and views of elite competitors. London: Sports Council, 1995.

29. Scarpino V, Arrigo A, Benzi G, Garattini S, La Vecchia C, Bernardi LR, et al. Evaluation of prevalence of "doping" among Italian athletes. *Lancet* 1990;336:1048–50.

30. Lombardo J. Drug control programmes. *Br J Sports Med* 1996;30:82–3.

8

Mandatory Drug Fest in Sports: The War Against Drugs Is Failing on All Fronts

Luke Cyphers

Luke Cyphers is a sports writer for the New York Daily News.

Drug testing, the main tool of the war on drugs in sports, fails to catch cheaters, erodes privacy rights, and sometimes unfairly tars honest competitors with drug abuse allegations. In elite sports, athletes who take recreational or performance-enhancing drugs will always find a way to cheat the drug tests. Testing in sports sets disturbing precedents for intruding on the privacy of others, including children.

With drug stories popping up across the playing fields like mushrooms after a summer rain, from tennis to football to track and field to Yankee Stadium, it's time to acknowledge some ugly truths.

In one form or another, everybody in sports takes drugs.

Further, the sports world's war against drugs has turned into Vietnam, and the war's main weapon, the drug test, is doing more harm than good, not catching real cheaters, wrongfully disgracing honest competitors and eroding privacy rights across the country.

Let's review.

- In the NFL, it was revealed that 16 players who tested positive for illegal street drugs or steroids in 1995 had their cases put "in abeyance" until a new labor agreement was reached. The league put a good spin on what looked like an inconsistent policy, saying the 16 cases were all grandfathered in under new rules, that no one "looked the other way." Later in the week, Denver linebacker Bill Romanowski, his wife and his doctor acknowledged being under investigation for drug fraud for improperly obtaining Phentermine, a weight-loss drug that can be used as speed.
- At the U.S. Open, sanctions against Petr Korda were upheld by an

international arbitration agency. Korda tested positive for the steroid nandralone, was banned, and successfully appealed to an independent panel. The panel sided with his argument that he did not know how he ingested the drug, but that decision was overturned.

- At Yankee Stadium, Darryl Strawberry came back to play after another bout with drug problems, which, incidentally, weren't discovered during his drug-testing program.

- In track, sprinter Dennis Mitchell described in a published report the nightmare he's had since failing track's now controversial testosterone-epitestosterone ratio test. Mitchell's testosterone levels were unnaturally high, according to the sport's rules. Mitchell's defense—which a noted endocrinologist found plausible—reads like something from the Starr Report. He drove all night, drank eight beers and had sex several times with his girlfriend, all of which drove his hormone levels higher than a 14-year-old at a Jennifer Lopez concert.

    Too much information, more than anyone who runs around in a playsuit for a living should be forced to divulge. But a desperate Mitchell was left with no other choice in an attempt to win an argument with a vial of urine.

- In Lewis Center, Ohio, it was business as usual for student-athletes at the Olentangy school district, who gave urine samples—a requirement for them to compete. Almost no one tested positive last year, and athletes do drugs less frequently than other students, says Joseph Franz, whose Sport Safe Testing Service runs the district's program. The district doesn't test for steroids, by the way. Too expensive.

Meanwhile, a thriving counter-industry markets products to beat the tests, including a compound peddled by comedian Tommy Chong—of "Up in Smoke" fame—called Urine Luck.

In most elite sports, testing seems pointless, because the cheaters will always find a better chemist than the urine police. The NFL spends "several million dollars" on its drug program, says league spokesman Greg Aiello, and its cooperation with the players in terms of getting them counseling and treatment before punishing them is laudable. But the policy didn't stop the Cowboys' "white house" shenanigans. Police did.

In most elite sports, testing seems pointless, because the cheaters will always find a better chemist than the urine police.

Policies don't mean public-relations points, either. The NBA was burned by reports about Reggie Lewis' death, which may have been due to cocaine, that indicted the league policy—once lauded as "the best in sports"—as a joke.

Craig Masback, the head of USA Track and Field, gets headaches when "blowhards on the Sports Reporters," as he calls them, talk about track being a dirty sport. "Our sport has been testing since 1960, and testing out of competition for 10 years, and guess what, we actually catch people," he says. "I guess we're stupid, but I think the people who are actually trying to do something should get applause."

What track gets is ignored until the Olympics.

In the U.S., the testing issue is further clouded by the country's horrible 1994 nutrition-supplement law, which allows androstenedione—which is sometimes spiked illegally with testosterone—to be sold to 10-year-olds at "health" stores.

Drug testing in sports has become a trojan horse eradicating privacy rights.

The NFL Players Association is formally warning players that it believes legal supplements have caused players to fail tests. "They think if it's over-the-counter, it's OK," says Stacy Robinson of the NFLPA. "But it's unregulated. The worst thing Congress did was that law (which was sponsored by Utah Sen. Orrin Hatch). Thanks Orrin."

All these are reasons to think about ditching drug tests, though it's not a popular idea. Masback, Aiello and Robinson all think systems can be improved, despite a long history to the contrary.

So does Joseph Califano, the former secretary of health, education and welfare and now head of Columbia's National Center on Addiction and Substance Abuse. "We are not going to drug test our way out of our problems," he says. "But like it or not, athletes are role models."

That applies to drug testing, too. Perhaps the worst aspect of the drug-test craze has been its trickle-down effects. Testing in sports sets frightening precedents for the rest of society, allowing self-appointed body police an excuse to put thousands of American children through urine tests as a prerequisite to playing on school teams.

It's a growing business, and many drug testing advocates don't want to stop at athletes. Says Joseph C. Franz, who runs a company that performs drug tests on athletes at Olentangy, Ohio, "Everybody would like to do the whole student body." So far, the courts haven't allowed it.

Drug testing in sports has become a trojan horse eradicating privacy rights. In some school districts, the tests have led to humiliating strip searches of teenage girls. School sports policies have also forced kids to reveal all prescriptions they take for medical conditions—even those that have nothing to do with their ability to play. Don't want your coach to know you take Ritalin? Too bad.

In America, games, it seems, are more important than the Fourth Amendment, the right to be left alone, or the right to keep medical issues private.

People like Califano, Masback and Robinson mean well when they defend drug testing. They believe athletes are heroes rather than mere entertainers. They're not. Big companies see athletes as programming, little different than Robert Downey Jr. or Janis Joplin or Mighty Mouse. So should the rest of us.

Athletes can still set examples about drug use, just like movie stars and rock stars have.

Cocaine killed the career of David Thompson, and stunted those of Darryl Strawberry and Dwight Gooden. Steroids killed the Raiders' Lyle Alzado, rotted Steeler Steve Courson's heart. Speed turned former Charger Walt Sweeney's life into a mess.

Retell those stories to young athletes, and you'll have an effective drug-prevention program. Those smart enough to get the message will stay off the stuff. Those stupid enough to do drugs will do them anyway, testing or no.

Remember this: The greatest drug casualty of them all, Len Bias, passed all his drug tests before being taken in the first round of the 1986 NBA draft. A few days later, he died of a cocaine overdose.

9

Athletes Have the Right to Accept the Risks and Benefits of Performance-Enhancing Drugs

Robert Lipsyte

Robert Lipsyte is a New York Times *sports columnist and the author of several books including* Idols of the Game: A Sporting History of the American Century.

At a time when many people are using drugs such as Prozac and Viagra to enhance their performance in the workplace and elsewhere, the distinction between necessary therapy and unethical performance enhancement has become harder to maintain. Athletes should not be held to a higher standard than the rest of society when it comes to using chemical substances to improve their performance. Drug testing procedures and other measures to control drug use are in part a battle for control over the sports industry between athletes and those who manage and profit from sporting events.

A thletes have always been contemptuous of sport's attempts to regulate drug use, but they tended to keep their mouths shut. Most resented the whip hand that testing gave management, but they were too afraid of being caught, punished, embarrassed to speak up unless they were squeaky clean, retired or busted.

Until last week [July 1998], when bicycle racers briefly disrupted the Tour de France as a protest against what they claimed was a witch hunt, athletes have never so publicly and boldly stood up to drug testing.

One knee-jerk reaction to the slowdown in the Alps was that the inmates were taking over the asylum, another that the so-called athletes' re-

Reprinted from Robert Lipsyte, "Competition and Drugs: Just Say Yes," *The New York Times*, August 2, 1998. Reprinted with permission from *The New York Times*.

volt had begun again after 30 years of simmering. A day later, the race continued, probably a tribute to favors and deals. But that little mountain uprising may yet turn out to be a historical turn in the road: athletes are finally expressing justified disgust with a capricious system that seems to be, in these days of what the University of Texas professor John Hoberman calls "the therapeutic ideal," simply out of date.

If drugs like Prozac and Viagra can be taken without apology by everyday people who want to enhance their performance in a competitive world, why shouldn't athletes, prized as models of "human capacity," be allowed, nay, encouraged, to try out drugs for the rest of us?

Unfair drug testing

Drug testing has not been fair—few marquee names have ever been brought down—nor as effective a deterrent as both sides would have fans believe. Athletes have gone along with the lie as long as it kept reporters from snooping around their specimens. Also, athletes have tended to stay ahead of the drug police.

As the rewards for victory have spiked, a growing network of underground pharmacologists have concocted drugs too new to be detected in addition to masking agents for the old drugs. This competitive cat-and-mouse game, risky, expensive and hypocritical, has allowed athletes to continue seeking the edge while management kept the appearance of control.

That game began unraveling along with the Tour last Wednesday [July 29, 1998]. When word reached the 140-rider pack that the police had raided a team's hotel and forcibly tested riders' urine, hair and blood for drugs, cyclists slowed down, quit, tore off their numbers, canceling the day's race.

By Thursday, with a half a dozen teams out of the competition, some 101 of the 198 riders who started on July 11 in Dublin were again rolling toward Paris and $2.2 million in prizes. Apparently, the most consistent performance enhancing drug is still money.

Nevertheless, two interlocked issues, one about control and the other about appropriate drug use, were once again out of the bottle.

Shouldn't athletes, prized as models of "human capacity," be allowed, nay, encouraged, to try out drugs for the rest of us?

Not since the 1960's, when Harry Edwards, Tommie Smith and John Carlos used the Olympics as a platform against racism; Muhammad Ali used the heavyweight championship as a pulpit; and Billie Jean King led tennis players—eventually all players—out of the desert of sham amateurism, have athletes rebelled so dramatically against management.

Current labor skirmishes, including the [1998] N.B.A. lockout, can also be seen in that context. The testing for drugs, recreational or performance enhancing (another distinction that is blurring), has always been the most subtle and insidious way of enforcing that control.

And just last Monday [July 27, 1998], two American Oympians—the sprinter Dennis Mitchell and the shot-put champion Randy Barnes—were suspended for possible doping offenses. Mitchell reportedly tested above the acceptable levels of testosterone.

On Friday [July 31, 1998], Barnes' B sample turned out positive, too, showing a banned nutritional supplement, androstenedione, a naturally occurring substance in the body that is available in health food stores.

Doping in sport and in life

The most significant incident, however, may have occurred four years ago [in 1994] when the marathoner Alberto Salazar ended a long streak without a victory. With the help of the antidepressant Prozac, which he was using legally as a training aid, he won the 56-mile Comrades Marathon in South Africa.

For the ever-provocative Hoberman, who wrote "Mortal Engines: The Science of Performance and the Dehumanization of Sport" in 1992, Salazar's drug of choice "forged a high-profile link between doping in sport and the wider world of pharmacology that affects us all."

Hoberman expects that "pharmacological Calvinism" will be increasingly harder to enforce in sports as drugs are "gentrified." In particular, he thinks that as more elderly men, and even women, use testosterone to enhance their lives, it will become impossible to prohibit the drug from enhancing sports performance.

The [1998] Tour ends in Paris today, and the current controversy may get a flat tire; only the squeaky clean, the retired and the busted will want to talk. But the struggle for control will continue in sports, as will the hypocrisy of drug testing.

The real issue for the future will be the legalization of drugs that cross the artificial line between therapy and performance enhancement. Hoberman's vision includes Olympians at the starting blocks, "their drug company logos gleaming in the sun."

10

Banning Performance-Enhancing Drugs Is Justified

Steve Olivier

Steve Olivier teaches at Staffordshire University in Great Britain.

Athletes should be prohibited from taking performance-enhancing substances such as stimulants and steroids because these drugs can harm those who use them. Although some would argue that a person has a right to choose whether to risk harm to one's own body, the use of drugs in sports can place athletes in a situation in which they feel coerced into taking drugs in order to compete. In addition, society has an interest in preventing the violence associated with the use of steroids and other drugs.

The use of drugs by athletes is not a new phenomenon, but in the last decade or so the issue has received much public attention. This has resulted in a renewed focus on the question of whether the use of performance-enhancing substances in sport ought to be prohibited. (We need to be aware of the distinction between the question of whether it is wrong to use performance-enhancing substances in sport, and the question of whether the use of these substances in sport ought to be prohibited. Prohibition does not necessarily follow from "wrongness.") In this paper I will argue that a certain class of performance-enhancing substances should be banned. In doing this, I shall first define performance-enhancing substances and then focus on arguments concerning self-harm and harm to others. The notions of coercion and subtle pressure will be examined, and this will serve as an attempt at justifying paternalism.

If one were to ask the proverbial "man in the street" whether the use of performance-enhancing substances in sport ought to be banned, it is likely that the majority of responses would be affirmative. If one were then to ask why, the answer would probably be justified by one of two lines of reasoning. Reason A would be that it is cheating, and this is contrary to the nature of sport. Reason B would be that the use of performance-enhancing

Reprinted from Steve Olivier, "Drugs in Sports: Justifying Paternalism on the Grounds of Harm," *American Journal of Sports Medicine*, November/December 1996. Reprinted with permission from *American Journal of Sports Medicine*.

substances should be prohibited because it is a harmful practice.

Argument A contends that sport is a valued human practice and, in terms of the ethos that characterizes it as such, the use of performance-enhancing substances is not only illegal (in terms of constitutive, regulative, and auxiliary rules), it is also morally reprehensible in that it violates the virtues of honesty and trustworthiness, which go to the heart of the fairness and integrity of competitive sport. In this paper I will not follow this line of reasoning but will instead evaluate those arguments supporting a ban on performance-enhancing substances that are underpinned by the notion of harm to one's self and others (Argument B).

Performance-enhancing substances defined

What exactly are we referring to when we talk about performance-enhancing substances? Very generally, we can initially group them as follows.

1. Stimulants (amphetamines, caffeine, cocaine, other sympathomimetic drugs).

2. Anabolic-androgenic steroids (synthetic derivatives of the male sex hormone testosterone).

3. Human growth hormone.

4. Erythropoietin.

(Note that for the purpose of this paper, the above grouping excludes narcotic analgesics, alcohol, marijuana, tobacco, and miscellaneous drugs such as beta-blocking agents, diuretics and nutritional supplements.)

Time does not permit an examination of the possible harmful effects of performance-enhancing substances. Let us, however, tentatively accept Wagner's conclusion that ". . . whether the ergogenic effects are real or perceived, the potential for adverse effects exists for all of these drugs. Potential health complications represent a serious risk to an otherwise healthy population."[1]

With regard to the ergogenic effects, the question of whether performance-enhancing substances produce meaningful changes in performance is much debated. Such debate is beyond the scope of this paper, which assumes that at the very least athletes who use these substances believe that ingestion will result in improved performance.

We must then make two assumptions for the discussion to proceed. The first is that performance-enhancing substances carry the risk of significant harm to the user, and the second is that use of these substances will significantly improve performance. With these assumptions in place, let us return to the primary question of the moral justification of prohibition by governing sports bodies. In other words, what are the moral underpinnings for not permitting individuals to pursue excellence by any means they choose?

Paternalism, coercion, choice, and harm to others

Earlier it was noted that one frequently advanced argument against the use of performance-enhancing substances refers to the potential risk for significant harm to the user. Quite simply then, this argument contends that since the use of performance-enhancing substances is harmful to the user, it ought to be prohibited. This is viewed as unjustified paternalistic inter-ference by some sports libertarians who would contend "It's my life, my body, and I should be at liberty to do with it whatever I want to, as long as I don't harm others." The qualification of not harming others, proponents of this view believe, renders their position consistent with [John Stuart] Mills' "harm principle." (Mill's Harm Principle states that the only purpose for which people may be coerced by law is to protect others from harm that they would, if not coerced, be inflicting on them.) This paper, however, ar-gues that use of performance-enhancing substances contributes to a situa-tion where others are potentially placed at risk.

In evaluating what I will call the "coercion argument," the central question that needs to be considered is whether athletes freely choose to ingest performance-enhancing substances, or whether they are in some way coerced to do so. (Here I will ignore direct coercion such as pressure from coaches and others and will focus on more subtle, but perhaps no less powerful, coercive agents). On the surface, it would seem that ath-letes can choose freely, but what about the pressures created by the need for success in competition? I am not just referring to the satisfaction of winning—rather, I am recognizing that in professional sports one's future may depend on winning. At this level, sports is one's means of employ-ment, and the greater the incentives to succeed, the greater the tempta-tion to use any method available to achieve that end. The pressure may thus be greater than some mere primeval satisfaction of the will-to-win.

Use of performance-enhancing substances is wrong not only because it harms the user, but because it may harm others as well.

Are athletes really not able to act and choose freely with regard to performance-enhancing substances? It could be argued that they are not forced to earn their living through sports. They, in fact, have the choice to follow a different vocation, for example, medicine or plumbing. Of course an athlete could choose a different career path, but the reality of the situation is not that clear-cut. Having devoted most of his or her life to the pursuit of excellence in athletics, the athlete is now confronted with the choice of taking a banned substance and remaining competitive or declining such use and entering the job market with precious little skill or experience. The choice is thus complicated because the athlete does not have the means to make it worthwhile, and we need to question whether it is realistic to expect this athlete to choose the nondrug route. Paternalism in this case is defended on the grounds that the athlete's cir-cumstances are such that it would be unreasonable to expect him or her to resist the pressure of the situation.

A further form of subtle coercion or influence is that of role models. Hero worship can be a powerful influence to act, and if an impressionable young athlete perceives that success is only attainable through a particu-lar practice, such as use of performance-enhancing substances, then the practice, which may be harmful to the role model, becomes potentially harmful to others. The recent case of the 14-year-old South African athlete Liza De Villiers, who, in April 1995, tested positive for nandrolone decanoate (an anabolic steroid) and fencamfamine (a stimulant) serves to illustrate that use of performance-enhancing substances is not only pervasive in adult sport, but that the practice may be common at junior levels. Schwellnus et al.[2] and Skowno[3] reported significant use of anabolic-androgenic steroids among schoolchildren involved in sports. If such usage can be linked to subtle (albeit unintentional) coercion, then the paternalist position is strengthened.

Essentially, the coercion argument holds that athletes who use performance-enhancing substances harm not only themselves, but that they contribute significantly to the creation of a climate that places some stricture on choice. One can choose: either be moral with regard to performance-enhancing substance use, perhaps to the detriment of your career, or disregard the ethics of the situation to perhaps ensure your future. So there is choice, but the element of coercion remains because the choice is difficult and the issues are not necessarily clear. If we accept this argument, use of performance-enhancing substances is wrong not only because it harms the user, but because it may harm others as well.

It seems justifiable to prohibit use of a substance if
. . . such use can lead to violent situations where
persons are harmed.

Further support for this coercion theory may be found outside the strictly competitive arena; again, I use research into steroid use as an example. Crist et al.[4] administered relatively high doses of testosterone cypionate and nandrolone decanoate to nine volunteer subjects to determine the effects of anabolic-androgenic steroids on neuromuscular power and body composition. Although no statistically significant effects were noted in this particular study, the subjects reported subjective feelings of increased strength after the administration of anabolic agents. Our coercion theory would hold that these subjective impressions may result in some sort of psychologic dependence to improve either performance or self-image, with the immediate effects being readily visible while the longer-term adverse effects are not apparent. In the first case then, pressures created by the nature of professional sports coerce subjects into use of performance-enhancing substances, and in the second case, such coercion is achieved by placing research subjects a step closer to temptation and, in so doing, creating a climate conducive to psychologic dependence.

Leaving coercion and competitive sport aside briefly, let us focus narrowly on specific possibilities of cases of harm to others where steroid use is involved. Some evidence now suggests that increased aggression is associated with steroid use. In a recent study, Choi and Pope[5] investigated physical abuse of significant others by steroid users. They state that their findings support the claims that partners of steroid users may be at risk of violence from users while they are "on-drug," and that steroid-associated violence toward other individuals may be more common than originally suspected.

The findings of the previously mentioned study strongly suggest that steroid use may be associated with increased aggression and violence. This is well established, with steroid use even being advanced as a contributory factor in lawsuits concerning violent crime. It seems reasonable to assume that steroid use by athletes could therefore contribute to on-field violence, particularly in sports such as rugby or football, where participants are (for a variety of reasons) predisposed to act and react aggressively. In such situations, the possibility of direct harm to others clearly exists.

Drug prohibition is justified

If we paternalistically deprive someone of a freedom (to use performance-enhancing substances), we need to justify this violation of autonomy by balancing the evil we hope to prevent against the loss of freedom we are advocating. In performing the sort of "moral accounting" described here, it is my contention that prohibition on the grounds of indirect harm to others (through coercion) is justified. "Soft" paternalists argue that limitations on liberty are justified when behavior is not fully voluntary because the person is not fully informed (e.g., as to the likely consequences of one's action), or because one is not fully competent or is being coerced in some relevant way. Given the coercion argument outlined above, the last condition is of course crucial to my justification for paternalistic interference, even in the difficult case of rational, informed, emotionally mature adults. Finally, it seems justifiable to prohibit use of a substance if a substantial body of research supports the contention that such use can lead to violent situations where persons are harmed.

I have examined some of the issues surrounding the banning of performance-enhancing substances in sports. In deliberately ignoring what I have called the "nature-of-sports" argument, and focusing on the notion of harm, I have argued that prohibition of harmful practices is justified by potential harm to others (rather than just to one's self). One must bear in mind the powerful effects of subtle coercion and influence and the consequent limitations placed on choice. So, on the grounds that it is wrong to harm others or to coerce them into potentially harmful situations, this paper takes issue with sports libertarians who claim that banning performance-enhancing substances is an unjustified paternalistic action that violates the principle of autonomy.

References

1. Wagner, J.C., "Enhancement of Athletic Performance with Drugs: An Overview," *Sports Medicine*, 12:250–265, 1991.

2. Schwellnus, M.P., Lambert, M.I., Todd, M.P., et al., "Androgenic Anabolic Steroid Use in Matric Pupils," *South African Medical Journal,* 82:154–158, 1992.

3. Skowno, J., "Drug Survey Among First Team Schoolboy Rugby Players," *South African Medical Journal,* 82:204, 1992.

4. Crist, D.M., Stackpoke, P.J., Peake, G.T., "Effects of Androgenic-Anabolic Steroids on Neuromuscular Power and Body Composition," *Journal of Applied Physiology,* 54:366–370, 1993.

5. Choi, F.Y.L., Pope, H.E., "Violence Towards Women and Illicit Anabolic-Androgenic Steroid Use in Strength Athletes," *Journal of Sports Science,* 12(2):184–185, 1994.

11

The United States Must Spearhead Reforms to Eradicate Drugs in Sports

Barry R. McCaffrey

Barry R. McCaffrey, a retired U.S. Army general, was appointed by President Bill Clinton to be director of the Office of National Drug Control Policy in 1996.

Drug use in sport has reached crisis levels, both among elite athletes and America's young people. A new strategy is needed to prevent drug use in the Olympics and in other sports. The United States government should take the lead in the fight against drugs in sports.

Editor's note: The following viewpoint is taken from Barry R. McCaffrey's testimony on drug use in sports before the Senate Committee on Commerce, Science, and Transportation on October 20, 1999.

From the "Miracle on Ice" to Dan Jansen's gold medal win dedicated to the memory of his sister, sports inspire us all to try harder and be better. As parents—and as a nation—we rely upon athletics to help us nurture healthy, strong children and to inculcate important values. For example, according to the Department of Health and Human Services, a child who plays sports is 49 percent less likely to get involved with drugs than a peer who does not play sports.[1]

However, these positive aspects of sport are now at risk to drug use and doping. Drug use and doping in sport has reached a level where athletes increasingly believe that they cannot compete honestly and win—chemical engineering is now perceived as a *sine qua non* to success.

Why drugs threaten sports

Drug use deprives honest athletes of a lifetime of hard work and dedication. Shirley Babashoff won six silver medals behind East German swimmers.

Excerpted from Barry R. McCaffrey, testimony before the Senate Committee on Commerce, Science, and Transportation, October 20, 1999.

When she raised questions about doping by the East German medal winners, the press unfairly denigrated this superb athlete of such enormous integrity. Subsequently, newly opened *Stasi* files made public through a series of lawsuits show that the former East German sports machine doped thousands upon thousands of athletes, many of whom were unwitting children—including Ms. Babashoff's competitors. To date nothing has been done to redress this extreme injustice.

Doping in sport has reached a level where athletes increasingly believe that they cannot compete honestly and win.

Every great victory is questioned. Track legend Edwin Moses and wrestling hero Bruce Baumgartner—both of whom compete cleanly and are leaders in fighting drug use—have spoken out about the anguish and loss of dignity they feel when total strangers approach them and ask if their honest victories were the product of doping. Even the 1999 Tour de France victory of Lance Armstrong, who came back from cancer, has been doubted. At base, doping has become so widespread that the many athletes who compete and win based solely on talent and determination are still viewed with skepticism.

America's youth are at risk. The threat of doping affects not just a few elite athletes, but millions of American children at all levels who dream of Olympic gold and other sport victories—from little league baseball to youth soccer to high school swimming. This threat occurs not just at the world class level, but in our own neighborhoods and schools.

- In 1998, a survey of Massachusetts youth reported in the well-respected journal *Pediatrics* found that 3 percent of girls ages 9 to 13 have used steroids.[2] Use among boys was found to be just under 3 percent. This is the first time that the use of steroids among girls was found to surpass use among boys. For both boys and girls, these levels are on par with use of other drugs of abuse. For example, the 1997 National Household Survey found that lifetime cocaine use by children ages 12–17 was 3 percent.
- The Healthy Competition Foundation's 1999 survey found that 1-in-4 young people personally know someone using performance enhancing substances. Knowledge grows substantially with age—9 percent of 12-year-olds personally know someone doping, compared with 32 percent of those ages 15–16 and 48 percent of those ages 17 and older.[3]
- The majority of young people report that steroids are easily available through their friends and their coaches.[4]

The threat of drug use in sports is growing. Our National Drug Control Strategy is producing real progress in reducing overall youth drug use. According to the 1998 National Household Survey, overall youth (age 12 to 17) drug use is down 13 percent from the previous year. Among this critical age group cocaine use is down 20 percent and inhalant use is down 45 percent over the same period. However, in sharp contrast, research indicates that today's highly competitive athletic world is causing youth performance enhancing drug use to grow significantly.

- According to the Monitoring the Future survey, the rate of steroid use among twelfth grade girls jumped 100 percent from 1991 to 1996. During this same period, steroid use among 10th grade females jumped 83 percent, and 75 percent among 8th grade females.
- Makers of Androstenedione (Andro) self-report that Andro sales are up roughly five-fold since last year.[5] (Andro, currently classed as a food supplement, is believed by many to improve performance. The Drug Enforcement Administration (DEA) is engaged in a scientific process to determine if Andro actually produces muscle growth—and, in turn, whether it should be classed as a steroid.)

Drug use in sports is now widely perceived as a public health crisis. The performance enhancing drugs now being used by increasingly younger and younger children put lives and health in real jeopardy. The American people recognize these risks and want them ended.

- According to a 1999 survey by the Healthy Competition Foundation, 75 percent of American adults see drug use and doping in sport as a public health problem.[6]
- This survey also found that 83 percent of American teens and preteens and 86 percent of adults disapprove of current drug use and doping in sport.[7]

Drug use in sports is now widely perceived as a public health crisis.

Performance enhancing drugs put the health and safety of those who use these substances at serious risk. These risks are particularly high for young people; the use of exogenous hormones during a child's development can seriously impair and/or alter the normal cycle of development. No victory is worth the damage these substances do to human health.

- The risks of steroid use include: elevated cholesterol levels; increased risks of heart disease; serious liver damage (e.g., blood-filled cysts and tumors); androgenizing of females (the irreversible development of male secondary sex characteristics by girls, including clitoral hypertrophy, breast atrophy and amenorrhea); behavioral changes, particularly heightened aggressiveness; and feminization of males (including shrinking of the testes, low sperm counts, the development of high-pitched voice and breast development).[8] Adolescents are also at risk of permanently stunting their growth.
- The adverse health impacts of performance enhancing drugs on athletes as documented in the German criminal doping trials have been devastating.[9] The files of the *Stasi* (the German secret police who ran East Germany's national doping program) clearly reflect these health horror stories in frightening detail.[10] *Stasi*-documented health problems include: Androgen-induced amenorrhea, severe ovarian cysts, advanced liver damage, and fetal malformation among pregnant women.[11]
- In the worst cases these drugs can even be deadly. The drug erythropoietin (EPO) is widely thought to have contributed to the

deaths of 18 Dutch and Belgian cyclists and 12 Scandinavian ori-
enteers in the late 1980s and early 1990s.[12] Documented incidences
of deaths related to the use of performance enhancing drugs go
back more than a century.[13]

*Trafficking in performance enhancing substances is a large and growing
criminal industry.*

- In the last year, the DEA has carried out a number of steroid investigations. In Dallas, authorities broke up a ring that smuggled
  steroids from Mexico for distribution to local gyms and high
  schools. In Pittsburgh, DEA agents worked with Thai counterparts
  to identify an international steroid ring that illicitly sold steroids
  over the Internet. In New York, the DEA arrested 15 members of a
  Russian organized crime group that reportedly smuggled more
  than two tons of anabolic steroids into the United States. The DEA
  is also conducting ongoing investigations of the importation of
  products labeled as androstenedione that actually contain steroids.
- According to the DEA, these and other investigations indicate that
  the international sale of steroids is becoming increasingly sophisticated and entrenched in criminal networks.

The need for a new anti-doping approach

Current anti-doping systems fail to provide athletes with the assurance
that a level playing field exists for those who do not want to cheat. Moreover, many athletes believe that the existing systems are public relations
tools, not effective counter-drug programs. Many athletes believe that
these systems are run in such a way as to catch unknown athletes—but
not stars or potential medallists.

Irregularities abound. The athletes, in general, completely lack confidence in the ability of the international community to prevent, detect
and punish drug use in sport. Moreover, the persistent pattern of irregularities in international competition raises serious doubts about the existing commitment of the International Olympic Committee (IOC) and the
international community to protect the interests of the vast majority of
honest athletes, the virtues of sport, and the health and safety of the competitors.

- At both the [1996] Atlanta and [1984] Los Angeles [Olympic]
  games the IOC Medical Commission failed to act on a series of positive drug test results among medal winners for banned substances.
  During the Atlanta Games only two positive samples were announced.[14] However, in an interview with the *London Sunday
  Times*, an internationally recognized expert who helped with the
  testing in Atlanta stated that "There were several other steroid positives from around the end of the Games which we [the lab] reported."[15] Lab officials subsequently reported that in each of these
  instances the samples were passed along to Prince de Merode, the
  Director of the IOC anti-doping program.[16] Prince de Merode has
  publicly stated that he discarded the samples for unstated "technical difficulties."[17] Neither the lab reports, nor the names of the athletes in question, nor the purported technical difficulties have ever
  been disclosed.

Structural flaws undermine existing anti-doping approaches.
- These problems exist not just at the world level, but here domestically. U.S. laws provide inadequate regulation over a range of performance enhancing drugs. Domestic sports, particularly professional sports, do not ban a number of substances that are banned in international competition. These conflicting regimes confuse athletes and the public and cause international concerns about U.S.-based anti-doping programs.
- Existing federal standards also require improvement. For example, a 1995 DOJ [Department of Justice]/DEA conference determined that "current provisions of the Federal Sentencing Guidelines establish grossly inadequate sentencing standards for steroid traffickers."[18]
- The current United States Olympic Committee (USOC) drug testing program has been able to achieve less than a 75 percent success rate in testing athletes out-of-competition—roughly one-quarter of the time, athletes who are selected for out-of-competition tests are not tested for logistical reasons (e.g., the athlete could not be found).[19] Yet, effective no-notice, out-of-competition testing is critical to any successful anti-doping regime.
- Moreover, the potential conflicts of interest that are inherent in our existing self-regulating approach have fueled international skepticism about the commitment of the United States to drug-free competition.

The essence of athletic competition is at risk. Recent drug scandals are without question eroding the ethical foundation of sport and are compromising the public's support for sport. A 1999 survey by the Healthy Competition Foundation found that 71 percent of the American people are less likely to watch the Olympics if they know athletes are using drugs. There is a growing perception that these games are becoming yet another fraud on the public.

Developing a new strategy

It is clear to the Office of National Drug Control Policy (ONDCP) that a new approach is required. With the health and safety of countless young people at stake and with the fate of one of the world's greatest tributes to the dignity of mankind in the balance, the Federal government has an obligation to play a role in creating such a solution. In the eloquent words of [track athlete] Edwin Moses:

> The problem of drug use by elite athletes must continue to be addressed on the Federal level by General McCaffrey and others who are responsible for children and the public welfare. . . . The United States is unique among Western democracies in not having a ministry of sport, because Americans generally believe that less government is good and that private organizations and the market can be trusted to do work that affects the public trust. Whatever the merits of this perspective in other contexts, the traditional deference to the private organizations that govern sport is not warranted in the case of doping. . . . Notwithstanding the efforts of some

well-intentioned individuals, the sports governing bodies in
this country and internationally have shown time and time
again that they are not structurally equipped for this work,
nor are they sufficiently accountable to the larger interests
of society that are affected by doping.[20]

Since the infamous Nagano snowboarding incident [in which a gold
medalist tested positive for marijuana during the 1998 Winter Olympics
in Nagano, Japan], the Office of National Drug Control Policy has been
examining the issue of drug use in sport. The result of these efforts is the
Strategy we are releasing today [October 20, 1999]. . . .

Key components of the national strategy

The Strategy begins from the understanding that the United States government has a responsibility to undertake efforts at the national, binational and international levels to strengthen anti-doping regimes. The
goals of these initiatives are to protect the health and safety of athletes
and young people and to safeguard the legitimacy of sports competition.
The Strategy also recognizes that to be effective these substantive initiatives should be augmented by efforts to inform the American public and
the international community about the risks of drug use in sport—as well
as the nature of our actions and goals.

Our Strategy provides a comprehensive set of national efforts to address this threat. We encourage you to review it in its entirety and welcome your views and leadership as we move forward. To assist you in this
review, this section highlights key elements of the Strategy.

1. National Efforts

Among the key initiatives at the national level are:

- *Developing options for targeted governmental oversight of U.S. amateur
  sports anti-doping programs.* An effective domestic anti-drug use program for sports may likely call for an oversight and reporting
  mechanism requiring Federal review and certification of amateur
  athletic anti-doping programs.

- *Working with the United States Olympic Committee (USOC) and other
  stakeholders to facilitate the development of an externalized and fully
  independent domestic anti-doping mechanism or body (including research, testing, and adjudication).* The development of an effective,
  transparent, accountable and independent U.S. agency is critical to
  the success of U.S. anti-doping efforts. Over the past year, the
  USOC has made significant strides toward building a more effective, transparent, independent and externalized anti-doping program. This effort is an important contribution to this Strategy.

In order to be effective, such an agency must be fully independent
and must have certain governmental or quasi-governmental powers. (For
example, the USOC has long sought membership in the International
Anti-Doping Arrangement (IADA). However, it has been precluded from
membership because the IADA is a treaty among governments and the
USOC is not a governmental body.) With the powers of governmental
status, however, must come the responsibilities of public service—most
notably the duties of transparency and accountability to the American

taxpayer. Further, an independent anti-doping agency would benefit substantially—both at home and abroad—from the added credibility offered by governmental oversight. Limited, but effective, oversight, accountability and transparency would allow the United States to dispel the perceived conflicts of interests and the "fox guarding the hens" reputation that unfortunately now plagues the program.

It is important to underscore that the purpose here is not to build a new government bureaucracy. Rather, the goal is to provide a level drug-free playing field for all of America's athletes, and to ensure that the institutions that police this field are effective, accountable and transparent. We look forward to working closely with the Congress and this Committee as we move forward in developing these institutions and relationships.

- *Improving Federal Support for U.S. Anti-Doping Programs.* From increasing drug prevention efforts to strengthening law enforcement operations to break up illegal smuggling networks, the Federal government should play a more active role in combating drug use in sport. The Strategy lays out a series of efforts that would support anti-drug and anti-doping efforts in the United States. The interagency task force will be evaluating ways to accomplish this goal.

One area where Federal support can be most valuable is in carrying out advanced research designed to end the "cat and mouse game" of current anti-doping programs by closing the existing scientific loopholes. Federally supported research has put a man on the moon and developed drug detection systems that can find a few ounces of drugs hidden within an entire truckload of produce. It seems nonsensical to suggest that we cannot find a way to determine if an athlete is chemically engineering his body.

- *Assisting the Salt Lake Games.* In 2002, the eyes of the world will turn to Salt Lake and the United States. Over the next two years, we have an important opportunity to set the standard for a drug-free Olympics. As the host nation it is our responsibility to ensure that we provide for the world's athletes a level playing field in Salt Lake. The Salt Lake Organizing Committee (SLOC) is committed to this goal. It is incumbent that we assist them in their efforts.

Current anti-doping systems fail to provide athletes with the assurance that a level playing field exists.

---

2. Binational Efforts—Australia and the United States

Our binational efforts focus upon building a partnership against drugs and doping between the Sydney and Salt Lake games. The anti-doping program being implemented for the Sydney games is impressive. For example, the Australians have also committed roughly $3 million to develop new drug testing and detection methods alone. Our goal in working with the Australians is to assist them as they prepare for the 2000 games and to learn from their efforts as we prepare for the 2002 games. The SLOC has already begun efforts in partnership with ONDCP to build such a team approach to combating doping—which is unheard of among host nations. Through effective teamwork, we have an opportunity to ensure that the last games of this millennium and the first games of the next millennium can begin a new drug-free era for the Olympic movement.

3. International Efforts

At the international level, our efforts are focused on achieving five commonsense principles within the world of international competition:

- A truly independent and accountable international anti-doping agency;
- Testing on a 365-day-a-year, no-notice basis;
- No statute of limitations—whenever evidence becomes available that an athlete cheated by doping they will be stripped of their honors;
- Deterrence through the preservation of samples for at least ten years—while a dishonest athlete may be able to defeat today's drug test, he or she has no way to know what will be detectable through tomorrow's scientific advances; and,
- Advanced research to end the present cat and mouse game of doping by closing the loopholes created by gaps in science.

Working with the IOC

These principles were first presented by ONDCP on behalf of the United States government to the IOC at the February, 1999 World Conference on Doping in Sport [in Lausanne, Switzerland].

Since the Lausanne meeting at which these markers were set out, the IOC has held a series of meetings to develop an anti-doping agency and program. The United States and the USOC were not included in these discussions—even though the United States is the largest market for the games, the bulk of the funding for the IOC and the games originates in the U.S. and we consistently field one of the largest teams in both summer and winter games. Nor were we consulted on the resulting text. Similarly, other nations—such as the Australians, the British, the Germans, the French and the Canadians—who are committed to the fight against drugs in sport were also not consulted. Of equal importance, only a few select athletes were part of this process.

As a result the IOC process has produced a proposal that does not meet the requirements we have set out. In general, it is our view that the IOC is rushing forward to build an institution that we cannot support—one which is more public relations ploy than public policy solution. Our central concerns include:

- The IOC's proposal provides the agency no real authority over anti-doping programs. Under the IOC's new Medical Code, anti-doping decisions of the agency would serve as mere recommendations to the IOC. This is not a model for either independence or effectiveness.
- The proposal should have stronger guarantees that the agency will be independent and operate based on basic principles of good governance and democracy, such as transparency and no conflicts of interest.
- The proposal asks national governments to pay half the bill for the agency, but fails to accord these governments a sufficient role in the policy-making process.
- Important decisions, such as the parameters of testing, have not

been addressed—instead they have been *de facto* delegated to a small executive board of IOC-related appointees to decide in secret.

With respect to funding, it seems inappropriate to assume that national governments will fund half the cost of an agency that they had no involvement in developing—and which they will have an inadequate role in operating. Further, while the international community should provide support for an adequate anti-doping agency of this sort, the "pay for a say" formula that has been set out fails to recognize that the nations hosting the upcoming games must also have a say in the agency—as is the case with the IOC's present Medical Commission. Additionally, the current IOC proposal fails to recognize the other contributions that many nations, such as the United States, have made and will make to the games—and the fight against drug use in sport.

We have once again consulted with many of our key partners, such as Australia, Canada and Great Britain. They continue to share the concerns that I have outlined. Further, while certain international organizations may have expressed agreement with the general direction of the IOC proposal, these organizations have not "endorsed" the IOC's proposal in the strict sense of the word (e.g., they have not taken it back to their member states for approval). Most importantly, the EU has informed us that during the discussions leading up to the IOC proposal, the EU made it clear that such a proposal could not appropriately move ahead without the involvement of the United States, the Australians, the Canadians and other national governments. These responses seem to refute the view expressed in public by IOC official Mr. Pound that the IOC's proposal has already been adequately endorsed internationally. However, we do have reason to believe that Mr. [Juan Antonio] Samaranch [president of the IOC] will be open to a reasonable discussion to achieve a rational consensus position.

Given this state of play, it is up to the international community to work with the IOC to ensure that an effective anti-doping regime is put in place. Ultimately, in order for any anti-doping regime to be effective, it must have the involvement of the international community, including the IOC, which is (rightly) a significant stakeholder in this effort.

Drug scandals are without question eroding the ethical foundation of sport.

ONDCP has begun efforts to develop an international consensus approach to rectify this situation. Over the coming months we will work closely with our U.S. stakeholders and international allies (e.g., the Australians, the Canadians, the British, the French, the Germans) and international organizations (e.g., the U.N. Drug Control Programme, and the Council of Europe) to develop such a consensus. This week [in October 1999], I will lead a U.S. interagency team to Europe to meet with our European allies. In November [1999], I will lead a delegation to a Summit of Governments on how to combat drug use in sports, which is being sponsored by the Australian government in Sydney.

Our purpose is to build a consensus sufficiently rational to bring the IOC to the table and require that these shortcomings be fixed. We look forward to helping the IOC work with the community of nations and the other stakeholders—in particular the athletes—to develop a truly independent and fully effective international anti-doping agency. We believe that the Australia Summit affords the IOC an important opportunity to move such a process ahead.

Mr. Chairman, knowing of your interest in this issue, we will keep you informed of developments on this front. If the IOC fails to seize this opportunity to work cooperatively with us and the rest of the international community, we will need your support to force change. In short, your leadership and that of the Committee will be critical to the creation of a truly independent agency and a fully effective international anti-doping regime.

Implementation of the national strategy

The Strategy before you is a living document. Between now and the 2002 games in Salt Lake the world of athletics—and the worlds of science and medicine—are likely to change dramatically. This Strategy provides a framework capable of evolving in parallel. In the near term we will convene the federal task force called for under the Strategy. This task force will be chaired jointly by ONDCP, the White House Olympic Task Force Chairs and HHS. This task force will include representatives from across the involved federal spectrum, including, but not limited to, the Office of Management and Budget, Justice (including DEA), State, the National Institute on Drug Abuse and the Substance Abuse and Mental Health Services Administration. The primary purposes of this task force will be to refine the Strategy, set priorities for implementation and undertake the task of implementing real reforms.

We believe that this should be an open and participatory process. We will reach out to the widest possible range of stakeholders—athletes young and old, coaches, doctors, the leaders of the National Governing Bodies, parents, sports organizations, and others. And, we will continue to work closely with the SLOC, USOC, and the USOC's Athletes Advisory Council—key actors in this effort.

Congressional leadership on sports issues has been strong. We recognize the important role that Congress plays in these matters. To this end, we will also seek out bipartisan Congressional representation on this task force and specifically look forward to working with the Chairman, Senator Hollings and this Committee.

The need for United States government leadership

Drug use in sports today has reached a level at which it jeopardizes both the integrity and legitimacy of athletics, as well as the health and safety of athletes and our youth. Athletes who want to compete fairly and without doping fear that they stand no chance against competitors who will accept any cost—debilitating injury, illness and even death—to win. Doping undermines the public trust in organized sport and the integrity of the vast majority of participating athletes who do not use drugs or dope. Every great victory is subject to doubt. Drug-using athletes verge on creating records that honest human performance cannot best. We seriously risk the creation of a chemically engineered class of athletic gladiators.

The current messages being sent by illicit, undetected, unreported or unresponded to drug use in sport continue to place our nation's young people at great risk. Each day, growing numbers of young people turn to untested and unproven chemicals to gain an edge. The age at which children—and in turn parents—are being confronted with the decision whether to use drugs or forgo them and face a competitive disadvantage is growing younger each year. Young people are confronted with the use of drugs, ranging from marijuana to steroids, among the ranks of elite athletes and consequently are led to the false belief that they can use drugs and succeed in life. At-risk youth are not limited to a few isolated elite athletes; on soccer fields, baseball diamonds and swimming pools all across the nation, hundreds of thousands of American children strive for greatness. Each of these young people are within the at-risk population.

First and foremost, doping control measures must be rooted in sports ethics and values. They must also be founded on respect for personal rights and the fairness of due process. Current doping and drug control programs have proven inadequate to the task. In general, they are limited in their ability to either effectively detect drug use or deter current or future athletes from cheating. Conflicts of interest—both real and apparent—abound. The current approach places honest athletes at risk of false accusations—and fails to ensnare those who actually cheat. Overall, today's systems fail to provide athletes with the assurance and confidence that the playing fields are level and that the clean competitors stand a fair chance at victory.

United States government leadership is critical if we are to succeed in eliminating the threat of drugs in sports.

Absent real reform, we risk not only irreparable damage to the beauty and glory of sports but also to the long-term health of our athletes and young people. Athletes willing to cheat will continue to push the envelope of science to find new ways to steal even the slightest advantage. Increasing numbers of ever younger children will acquiesce to the risks of drugs in order to pursue their athletic dreams. Absent change, the value of sports in our society will diminish and the human spirit will be poorer for its loss.

United States government leadership is critical if we are to succeed in eliminating the threat of drugs in sports. With such leadership, a strategy comprising national, binational and international efforts can help bring about needed reforms. Working with stakeholders (athletes, youth, the USOC (including the USOC Athletes Advisory Council), the NCAA, NGBs [national governing bodies], the leagues, coaches, doctors, parents, schools and others), we have an important window of opportunity to preserve the values of athletic competition and to safeguard the futures of our children.

Athletics at all levels play a major role in American society. Aside from their recreational value, we look to sports to help us as parents and as a nation to develop healthy children and instill positive values and mores in our youth. Feats of athletic greatness—the victory of the 1999 U.S. Women's World Cup soccer team, the U.S. hockey team's "miracle on ice," Jessie Owens' victories in the face of Nazism—inspire us and remind us to strive to be better in all that we do in pursuit of excellence. Athletics shape our culture, heritage and history. In this nation, sports provide us with rallying points around which diverse groups of people can unite and cheer with one voice. By working to safeguard sports we help preserve these important contributions to our nation.

Endnotes

1. *See* HHS, *Adolescent Time, Risky Behavior, and Outcomes: An Analysis of National Data* (September 1995); *see also* NFHS, *The Case for High School Activities* (undated) (available at www.nfhs.org) (discussing Hardiness Center study finding that roughly 92 percent of participants in high school sports were non-drug users, received above average grades and had better chances of attending and succeeding in college); T. Collingwood, *et al., Physical Fitness Effects on Substance Abuse Risk Factors and Use Patterns,* 21 J. Drug Education 73–84 (1991); E. Shields, *Sociodemographic Analysis of Drug-Use Among Adolescent Athletes: Observations—Perceptions of Athletic Directors-Coaches,* 30 Adolescence 839–861 (1995).

2. *See* A.D. Faigenbaum, et al., *Anabolic Steroid Use by Male and Female Middle Students,* Pediatrics, May 1998 (this survey was conducted in public middle schools in Massachusetts).

3. *Id.*

4. *See* S.M. Tanner, *et al., Anabolic Steroid Use by Adolescents: Prevalence, Motives, and Knowledge of Risks,* 5 Clin. J. Sports Med. 108–115 (1995). Fifty-five percent of young people report that steroids are easily attainable. *Id.* Friends and coaches were the two most often reported sources for these drugs. *Id.*

5. *See* Steve Wilstein, *Baseball Unlikely to Rule on Andro,* Associated Press, Feb. 27, 1999 (citing tenfold increase). The industry's own study noted a three-fold increase between the time of the McGwire revelation (August 1998) and December 1998 alone. *See* Steve Wilstein, *McGwire Powers Andro Sales to 100,000 Users, Doctors Fear Hazards,* Associated Press, Dec. 8, 1998.

6. Blue Cross/Blue Shield, Healthy Competition Foundation, Summary of Findings From National Surveys on Performance Enhancing Drugs, August 1999.

7. *Id.*

8. *See, e.g.,* Werner Franke, Brigitte Berendonk, *A Secret Governmental Program of Hormonal Doping and Androgenization of Athletics: The German Democratic Republic* (unpublished manuscript) (documenting health impacts on GDR athletes who used performance enhancing drugs); A.B. Middleman, *et al., Anabolic Steroid Use and Associated Health Risks,* 21 Sports Med. 251–255 (April 1996); S.M. Tanner, *et al., Anabolic Steroid Use by Adolescents: Prevalence, Motives, and Knowledge of Risks,* 5 Clin. J. Sports Med. 108–115 (1995); M.A. Nelson, *Androgenic-Anabolic Steroid Use in Adolescents,* 3 J. Pediatric Health Care 175–180 (Jul–Aug 1989); C.E. Yesalis, *et al., Anabolic Steroid Use Among Adolescents: A Study of Indications of Psychological Dependence,* in C.E. Yesalis, ed., Anabolic Steroids in Sport and

Exercise 215–229 (1993); C.E. Yesalis, *et al.*, *Anabolic-Androgenic Steroid Use in the United States*, 270 JAMA 1217–1221 (1993); M. Johnson, *et al.*, Steroid Use in Adolescent Males, 83 Pediatrics 921–924 (1989); K.E. Friedl, *Effects of Anabolic Steroids on Physical Health*, in C.E. Yesalis, ed., Anabolic Steroids in Sport and Exercise 109–150 (1993); R.H. Durant, et al. *Use of Multiple Drugs Among Adolescents Who Use Anabolic Steroids*, 328 N. Eng. J. Med. 922–926 (1993).

9. *See* Richard Panek, *Tarnished Gold*, Women's Sports and Fitness, May 1, 1999, 124. "Rica Reinisch, winner of three golds in 1980, blamed her ovarian cysts on hormones she'd taken. . . . Shot-putter Heidi Krieger, the 1986 European champion, contended that her unwitting ingestion of male hormones had led to facial hair, an Adam's apple and her eventual decision to undergo a sex change."

10. Werner Franke, Brigitte Berendonk, *A Secret Governmental Program of Hormonal Doping and Androgenization of Athletics: The German Democratic Republic*, 43 Clinical Chem. 1262–1279 (1997).

11. *Id.*

12. *See* Sean Fine, *et al.*, *Canadian Cyclist Watches Dream Die*, The Globe and Mail, Nov. 7, 1998; Dr. Gary Wadler, *Drug Abuse Update*, The Medical Clinics of North America, 439–455 (1994).

13. *See* G. Wadler and B. Hanline, Introduction, in *Drugs and the Athlete*, 1–17 (1989). In 1886, an English cyclist died from an overdose of the stimulant trimethyl. *See* Gary Wadler, *Doping in Sport: From Strychnine to Genetic Enhancement, It's a Moving Target*, presentation before the Duke Conference on Doping, May 7, 1999. In 1904, marathoner Thomas Hicks became the first death in the modern Olympics from the stimulant strychnine. *Id.* In 1960, Danish cyclist Knud Jensen died during the Rome Olympics from amphetamines. In 1967, English cyclist Tom Simpson died during the Tour de France. The autopsy revealed high levels of amphetamines. *See* E.M. Swift, *Drug Pedaling*, Sports Illustrated, June 5, 1999, at 65. Among the most egregious drug use practices reported by Mr. Voet, is the use of the so-called "Belgian cocktail"—a mix of amphetamines, cocaine, caffeine and heroin.

14. *See* John Hoberman, *SmithKline Beecham and the Atlanta Olympic Games* (unpublished paper on file at ONDCP).

15. *Id.;* Steven Downes, *Revealed: Four More Olympic Drug Users*, Sunday Times (London), Nov. 19, 1996.

16. *See Das Erbe von Atlanta: Vier vertusche Dopingfalle*, Süddeutsche Zeitung, Nov. 19, 1996; Hoberman supra n. 25.

17. *See supra* n. 16.

18. *See* U.S. Department of Justice, Drug Enforcement Administration, Conference on the Impact of National Steroid Control Legislation in the United States, June 1995.

19. John Powers, *Supplement User Striking Out*, Boston Globe, Sept. 6, 1998.

20. *See* Edwin Moses, *McCaffrey Must Not Stop at Andro*, New York Times, May 23, 1999, 13.

12

Drug Use in Sports Is Not Eradicable

Matt Barnard

Matt Barnard is a journalist and writer for the New Statesman.

While many people find the idea of using performance-enhancing drugs disturbing, athletes, responding to internal and external pressures to win and to improve, will continue to use them. Society will eventually accept the fact that elite athletes will use any means, including drugs, in their quest for success. Drugs will eventually be as accepted in sports as they are in medicine and cosmetics.

Florence Griffith Joyner ("Flo-Jo") died, aged 38, from heart seizure this week [September 1998]. Even before her untimely death, the shadow of suspicion hung over her glorious two gold medals and one silver at the Seoul Olympics in 1988: with her muscular form and husky voice typical of steroid users, and with her retirement announced abruptly in 1989, when mandatory random testing for drugs was introduced, there were whispers that Flo-Jo had used performance-enhancing drugs.

Flo-Jo's death will throw the spotlight back on to the debate over drugs in sports. Earlier this month another athlete was etching his name into the record books. The US baseball player Mark McGwire hit the most home runs ever in a single season, America's most prestigious sporting record. He is the first athlete in history to break a record while publicly admitting his use of performance-enhancing drugs. McGwire has admitted taking the drug androstenedione, which helps to build muscle and aids recovery from injury or exhaustion. The drug is on the banned list of the International Olympic Committee but is not banned by baseball's governing body, nor is it illegal. So far the use of drugs has not doomed baseball.

McGwire's chemically-aided race against the record book is credited with reviving interest in America's first game, giving it a renewed sense of value after the player strikes of 1994. As in many walks of life, unbridled success is able to sweep any latent moral misgivings neatly under the carpet.

Less predictably, however, the crowds lining the roads during this

Reprinted from Matt Barnard, "Drugs and Darwin Fuel Athletes," *New Statesman*, September 25, 1998. Reprinted with permission from Guardian News Service Ltd.

year's [1998] Tour de France applauded the cyclists as they swept past, supporting them despite the revelations of systematic drug-taking. The heavy-handed way the authorities conducted their investigation did little to win them support, and many spectators found it easy to empathise with athletes who had spent eight hours a day for two-and-a-half weeks slogging their guts out in one of the world's toughest competitions.

The moral crusade against the use of drugs in sport, like most moral crusades, is surrounded by myth. One of the myths is that fans won't pay to see drug-aided athletes perform, something that McGwire's example, and to a lesser degree the Tour de France, seem directly to contradict. It is said that more people turn up to watch McGwire warm up than attend most matches.

A second myth is that using drugs means that athletes don't have to work for their achievements. But, as Nicholas Pierce, lecturer in sport and exercise medicine at Queen's Medical Centre in Nottingham, comments: "Athletes will always be pushing themselves to the limit; if you could help push them further, they will go further."

The former cyclist Tommy Simpson is often mentioned in the context of sport and drugs, as he was one of the first athletes to die as a result of taking performance-enhancing stimulants. What commentators tend not to mention is that he literally worked himself to death. He pushed himself so hard that his heart gave out. Whatever one thinks about athletes who take drugs, they don't lack courage.

It is undoubtedly true, nonetheless, that the idea of using performance-enhancing drugs is deeply disturbing to a great many people. John Whetton is a former Olympic 1,500 metres finalist and European champion and is now a principal lecturer in life sciences at Nottingham Trent University. He is very clear that chemicals and sport shouldn't mix: "Using chemicals to do what your body isn't capable of doing is cheating, but it is a form of cheating that is hidden and therefore it is a nasty form of cheating."

But McGwire is open about his drug-taking, and as has become clear in the aftermath of this year's Tour, within cycling the use of drugs is an open secret.

Yet why are athletes who secretly do altitude training not tarred with the same brush? Clearly, the opposition to using drugs in sport is based on more fundamental assumptions than that it is simply not allowed by the rules.

A . . . myth is that using drugs means that athletes don't have to work for their achievements.

From the time the Greeks formulated the Olympic ideal, sport has held a more significant place in our culture than merely a leisure pursuit. In many ways it is used as a looking glass for the way we think about society. Richard Kerridge, co-editor of *Writing the Environment*, published earlier this year [1998], sees society's attitude to sport as being a web of concepts all entangled around the idea of what is "natural" and how we define "nature".

We see sport, he believes, as a celebration of nature, a way of demonstrating the wonders of creation, which is combined with the idea of dis-cipline, abstinence and purity. "In part," he says, "it's to do with the Christian tradition, in which to violate the laws of nature is to usurp the power of God. The taboo is about interfering in nature and interfering with the body." With such a background, it is not surprising that drugs are anathema.

On top of those ancient foundations is the more recent idea that sport is a form of capitalist competition. Kerridge says: "Characteristic of this attitude is that sport involves a relentless pressure for a kind of growth, so the standards always have to be pushed higher and higher."

The truth is that drugs are here to stay.

Though capitalism is based on the dog-eat-dog world of Darwinian survival, historians point out that the tradition of economic liberalism has always been combined with a strong sense of moral paternalism. It is perfectly acceptable to have obscene differences in wealth, but if a pauper is caught stealing a loaf of bread they should be publicly flogged. Simi-larly in sport, athletes and sporting nations may have hugely differing re-sources and expertise, but that is part of the free market of sport. How-ever, that free market has strict moral borders, and drug-taking falls outside them.

In order to reinforce that border, everyone involved in the "war on drugs" emphasises the physical risks involved. They are significant: liver failure and an increased chance of a heart attack are among the condi-tions associated with performance-enhancing drugs. Because of the ban on them, however, very little research has been done on how to reduce the risk.

The former Soviet states poured millions of pounds into developing performance-enhancing drugs, using the athlete as guinea pig—the indi-vidual as the servant of the collective. Nicholas Pierce is completely op-posed to the use of drugs in sport, but is forced to admit that with very large funds available it would be possible to develop a performance-enhancing drug that is virtually free of side-effects. And that, he argues, would have beneficial consequences for the rest of society: "It would be a tremendous boost for medicine as well. It would help people recover from operations and all sorts of things."

Athletes would become the equivalent of test pilots, who take high risks and sometimes get injured or killed. Unlike test pilots, though, at present there would be no safety checks or organisations to back them up. Indeed, many feel that sporting bodies and sponsors covertly encourage athletes to take drugs, yet abandon and condemn the few who get caught.

Michele Verroken, head of the Ethics and Doping Directorate at the UK Sports Council, has had direct experience of the lengths to which sports bodies will go to protect themselves. "It's not unusual," she says, "to have some of the major sporting organisations in this country asking us not to test athletes prior to a major sporting event like the Olympic or Commonwealth games."

Verroken, like many others, also raises questions about the drug-testing at the 1996 Atlanta Olympics, where the results went through organisations that had a direct interest in making sure the games were a commercial success, rather than through an independent testing organisation.

"In Euro 96, UEFA [Union of European Football Associations] worked very closely with us, so all the reports from the drug-testing process were reported through us. Is that what happened in Atlanta, or were the reports going straight back into the hands of the sports bodies who have a vested interest in making sure nothing clouds that event?

"It's not just an organisation like the International Olympic Committee, but it may be the organising committee from Atlanta or sponsors who pay an awful lot of money to have their name associated with the event and suddenly they are the 'whatever-company drug-infested games'. Those are the sorts of headlines that devastate the marketing people. Athletes feel they have been badly let down by the sports organisations that should have been protecting them."

One of the most surprising reactions to McGwire's achievement of breaking the record for home runs came from one of his teammates, who said: "What Mark has is God-given." It seems that in baseball the competitors have accepted that drug-taking is a legitimate training aid, but that it is only an aid.

The truth is that drugs are here to stay. Juan Antonio Samaranch, president of the IOC, had to back-pedal after he said that only drugs that harmed an athlete should remain on the banned list. But his was the first official brick to fall from the dam. We will accept drugs in sport—at elite level—just as surely as we accept them in medicine, cosmetics or farming.

Verroken's response to such an assertion is simple: "If a safe performance-enhancing drug improved everybody's performance to the same extent, what would be the point of taking it?" The answer is that, rightly or wrongly, every athlete has inscribed on their heart the words *citius altius fortius*—swifter, higher, stronger, as the Olympic motto reads. They will go to almost any lengths to push the barriers back.

Organizations to Contact

The editors have compiled the following list of organizations concerned with the issues debated in this book. The descriptions are derived from materials provided by the organizations. All have publications or information available for interested readers. The list was compiled on the date of publication of the present volume; the information provided here may change. Be aware that many organizations take several weeks or longer to respond to inquiries, so allow as much time as possible.

Canadian Centre for Ethics in Sport (CCES)
1600 James Naismith Dr., Suite 205, Gloucester, ON K1B 5N4 Canada
(613)748-5755 • fax: (613)748-5746
e-mail: info@cces.ca • website: www.cces.ca/english/drugfr0.html

CCES strives to promote drug-free sports in Canada and in international competitions. It produces and disseminates educational materials on performance-enhancing drugs and administers drug testing in Canadian athletic programs.

International Olympic Committee
Chateau de Vidy, CH-1007 Lausanne, Switzerland
fax: 011-41-21-621-6216
website: www.olympic.org

The IOC administers the Olympic Games. Its anti-doping code, updated in January 2000, prohibits the use of performance-enhancing drugs and maintains a list of banned substances. Its website includes information on banned substances, the World Anti-Doping Agency established in November 1999, and other related matters.

National Center for Drug Free Sport
810 Baltimore, Suite 200, Kansas City, MO 64105
(816) 474-8655 • fax: (816) 502-9287
e-mail: Info@drugfreesport.com
website: www.ncaa.org/sports_sciences/drugtesting/

The National Center for Drug Free Sport administers drug tests required by the National Collegiate Athletic Association. It can provide updated information on banned substances and drug testing procedures.

National Clearinghouse for Alcohol and Drug Information
PO Box 2345, Rockville, MD 20847-2345
(800) 729-6686 • fax: (301) 468-6433
e-mail: shs@health.org • www.health.org

The clearinghouse distributes publications of the U.S. Department of Health and Human Services, the National Institute on Drug Abuse, and other federal agencies. Publications include *Tips for Teens About Steroids* and *Anabolic Steroids: A Threat to Body and Mind.*

National Collegiate Athletic Association (NCAA)
6201 College Blvd., Overland Park, KS 66211-2422
(913) 339-1906
website: www.ncaa.org

The NCAA is the administrative body overseeing intercollegiate athletic programs. It provides drug education and drug testing programs. Information on its bylaws can be found on its website. The NCAA's publications include the *Guide for the College Bound Student-Athlete*.

National Strength and Conditioning Association
1955 N. Union, Colorado Springs, CO 80909
(719) 632-6722 • fax: (719) 632-6367
e-mail: nsca@usa.net • website: www.nsca-lift.org

The association seeks to facilitate an exchange of ideas related to strength development among its professional members. The association offers career certifications, educational texts and videos, as well as the bimonthly journal *Strength and Conditioning*, the quarterly *Journal of Strength and Conditioning Research*, and the bimonthly newsletter *NSCA Bulletin*. Its website includes an index of articles on ergogenic aids, including anabolic steroids.

OATH
1235 Bay St., Fourth Floor, Toronto, ON M5R 3K4 Canada
(877) 843-6284 • fax: (416) 534-7690
e-mail: oath@interlog.com • website: www.theoath.org

OATH is an independent international athlete-led organization that seeks to preserve the ideals of the Olympics, and to provide past and present Olympic athletes a united voice on doping and other issues. It has issued reports on Olympic reforms on anti-doping strategies.

Office of National Drug Control Policy
Executive Office of the President
Drugs and Crime Clearinghouse
PO Box 6000, Rockville, MD 20849-6000
e-mail: ondcp@ncjrs.org • website: www.whitehousedrugpolicy.gov

The Office of National Drug Control Policy is responsible for formulating the government's national drug strategy and the president's antidrug policy. It has worked to improve procedures for preventing drug use in sports. Drug policy studies are available upon request or at its website.

UK Sports Council
40 Bernard St., London, WC1N 1BR United Kingdom
011 020 7841 9500
e-mail: info@uksport.gov.uk • website:www.uksport.gov.uk

The UK Sports Council works to promote and support British athletes in world competitions and to promote anti-doping strategies and ethical standards in sports. Its publications include *Competitors and Officials Guide to Drugs and Sport*. More information is available on its website.

United States Olympic Committee (USOC)
One Olympic Plaza, Colorado Springs, CO 80909-5746
fax: 719-578-4654
website: www.usoc.org

USOC is a nonprofit private organization charged with coordinating all Olympic-related activity in the United States. It works with the International Olympic Committee and other organizations to discourage the use of drugs in sports. Information on its programs is available on its website.

Websites

Healthy Competition Campaign
www.healthycompetition.org

The website is part of a public education program launched by the Blue Cross and Blue Shield Association, a federation of health insurers, and provides information on performance-enhancing drugs for teens, parents, and coaches.

International Drugs in Sport Summit
http://drugsinsport.isr.gov.au/

This website includes information and papers presented at a November 1999 summit of government officials hosted by the Australian Minister for Sport and Tourism.

SteroidAbuse.org
www.steroidabuse.org

A service of the National Institute on Drug Abuse (NIDA), this website provides information and articles on the health risks of taking anabolic steroids.

Bibliography

Books

Charlie Francis — *Speed Trap*. New York: St. Martin's, 1990.

Bob Goldman and Ronald Klatz — *Death in the Locker Room: Drugs and Sports*. Chicago: Elite Sports Medicine, 1992.

Jeffrey Meer — *Drugs and Sports*. New York: Chelsea House, 1997.

Stan Reents — *Sports and Exercise Pharmacology*. Champaign, IL: Human Kinetics, 2000.

Kevin R. Ringhofer — *Coaches' Guide to Drugs and Sport*. Champaign, IL: Human Kinetics, 1995.

Ray Tricker and David L. Brown, eds. — *Athletes at Risk: Drugs and Sport*. Dubuque, IA: W.C. Coo, 1990.

Robert Voy with Kirk D. Deeter — *Drugs, Sport, and Politics*. Champaign, IL: Leisure, 1991.

Ivan Waddington — *Sports, Health and Drugs: A Critical Sociological Perspective*. New York: Routledge, 2000.

Melvin H. Williams — *The Ergogenics Edge: Pushing the Limits of Sports Performance*. Champaign, IL: Human Kinetics, 1997.

Charles E. Yesalis, ed. — *Anabolic Steroids in Sport and Exercise*. Champaign, IL: Human Kinetics, 2000.

Chalres E. Yesalis and Virginia S. Cowart — *The Steroids Game: An Expert's Inside Look at Anabolic Steroid Use in Sports*. Champaign, IL: Human Kinetics, 1998.

Periodicals

Natalie Angier — "Drugs, Sports, Body Image, and G.I. Joe," *New York Times*, December 22, 1998.

Michael Bamberger — "The Magic Potion," *Sports Illustrated*, April 20, 1998.

Sharon Begley and Martha Barnt — "The Real Scandal," *Newsweek*, February 15, 1999.

Ira Berkow — "FINA's Testing Is Marred, Too," *New York Times*, August 9, 1998.

Karen Birchard — "Why Doctors Should Worry About Doping in Sport," *Lancet*, July 4, 1998. Available from 655 Avenue of the Americas, New York, NY 10010 or at www.thelancet.com.

Philip M. Boffey — "Post-Season Thoughts on McGwire's Pills," *New York Times*, September 30, 1998.

Jane E. Brody — "The Muscle-Building Secret Is Out of the Bottle," *New York Times*, September 1, 1998.

David Brown — "Can 'Andro' Be Too Much of a Good Thing?" *Washington Post National Weekly Edition*, October 8, 1998. Available from 1150 15th St. NW, Washington, DC 20007.

Geoffrey Cowley and Martha Brant — "Doped to Perfection," *Newsweek*, July 22, 1996.

Karen Goldberg Goff — "Despite Sensitive Testing, Athletes Still Dope to Win," *Insight*, March 15, 1999. Available from 3600 New York Ave. NE, Washington, DC 20020.

Christine Gorman — "Muscle Madness," *Time*, September 7, 1998.

John W. Honour — "Testing for Drug Abuse," *Lancet*, July 6, 1996.

Derrick Z. Jackson — "McGwire Is Fooling Himself," *Liberal Opinion*, September 14, 1998. Available from PO Box 880, Vinton, IA 52349-0880.

Frederick C. Klein — "Drug Tester Needles the Olympics," *Wall Street Journal*, May 8, 1998.

Kathiann M. Kowalski — "Steer Clear of Steroid Abuse," *Current Health*, March 1999.

Jennifer Longley — "Hazard Alert," *People Weekly*, October 12, 1998.

E. Masood — "Performance-Enhancers Pose Dilemma for Rule-Makers," *Nature*, July 4, 1996. Available from reprints@natureny.com or at www.nature.com.

John Nicol — "Saying No to the IOC," *Maclean's*, February 15, 1999.

Holcomb B. Noble — "Questions Surround Performance Enhancer," *New York Times*, September 8, 1998.

Mike Penner — "Drug Bans, Suspicions Only Make Matters Worse," *Los Angeles Times*, August 20, 1999.

A. Pipe — "Drugs, Sport, and the New Millennium," *Clinical Journal of Sports Medicine*, January 2000. Available at www.cjsportmed.com.

Rick Reilly — "Hey, Mac, Do What Comes Naturally," *Sports Illustrated*, March 1, 1999.

William C. Rhoden — "Baseball's Pandora's Box Cracks Open," *New York Times*, August 25, 1998.

Skip Rozin — "Steroids: A Spreading Peril," *Business Week*, June 19, 1995.

Sports Illustrated — "Hockey's Little Helpers," February 2, 1998.

E.M. Swift — "Drug Pedaling," *Sports Illustrated*, July 5, 1999.

Phillip Whitten — "Strong-Arm Tactic," *New Republic*, November 17, 1997.

Christopher P. Winner — "Sports Doping Crisis Faces a Crossroads," *USA Today*, September 29, 1998.

Jason Zengerle — "Unspecial Olympics," *New Republic*, February 15, 1999.

Glenn Zorpette — "Andro Angst," *Scientific American*, December 1998.

Index